If It's Not Written Down,

It Never Happened!

Developing Critical EMS Reporting Skills

for Paramedics and EMTs

By Paul Serino M.ED, NRP

If It's Not Written Down,

It Never Happened!

Dedication

This book is dedicated to all EMS professionals who continuously strive to be better today than they were yesterday.

This sentiment was never better exemplified than by my two late friends, Ziggy and Randerson.

Thank you both for your service and showing me a person can make a full career working in EMS while maintaining a high standard of professionalism, humility and a wicked sense of humor!

I miss you both!

It's also dedicated to

All those who aren't always looking elsewhere to see where the grass is greener but instead work harder to see how they can make their own patch of lawn a nicer place to be.

I hope you enjoy it.

"You will find that many of the truths we cling to depend on our own point of view." -Obi Wan Kenobi (1983)

Introduction

Why Is Documentation So Unappreciated?

How can it be?

How is it the ability to write a strong Patient Care Report (PCR) is frequently considered to be one of the most undervalued skills we possess as EMS professionals?

This despite the fact it is one of the most consistently used skills in EMS?

Every patient interaction receives a PCR. **Every one!**

Critical, non-critical, interfacility, and scheduled patient transport all have details and demographics that are required to be documented. Each piece of information you choose to include or omit is a decision made by you to accurately detail the care and transport you provided during your time with a patient.

Heck, even patients we don't happen to transport, like refusals and patient transfers to other EMS services, like a medical helicopter, require a thoroughly documented PCR.

So, with this degree of frequency, one would think just by sheer repetition we would have mastered this particular skill, perhaps more than any other!

And yet the simple truth is, most of us still either don't feel confident writing a strong EMS report or simply do not value the importance of consistently being able to write a solid report despite doing it several times each shift.

Perhaps it's because we don't really think of writing as a skill. It's just something we are often forced to do at the end of a call. We don't stop to appreciate what it actually takes to produce a strong EMS chart that will stand up and not only give the reader a sense of what we saw throughout the call, but also why we chose the route of care we decided upon.

But why is this common problem? Is it that the reasons are visceral? To be sure we cannot always *see* the immediate effects of how a PCR is going to affect our patient's current condition. *But trust me, they do.*

Or is it something more tactile? We cannot touch and feel how our PCR plays into the patient's overall care the same way we can when performing a physical assessment or medical interventions.

And maybe, it's simply a fundamental lack of understanding as to how a PCR plays into the overall continuation of patient care that is to blame.

The subject of how to write a PCR is covered in both EMT and paramedic school, but the time spent on it is woefully brief. Usually a lecture, perhaps a skill review, and that's pretty much it.

The same can be said about the amount of documentation training a first responder received after they graduate and earn their patch.

How often are the benefits of writing a strong PCR covered in a refresher or lectured on at national or local conferences? *Here's a hint... not that often.*

By comparison, how much time did you spend in paramedic school studying pharmacology or cardiology? Or from a skills perspective, how many times did you practice inserting an IV or attempt to secure an ET tube?

Once?

Twice?

Perhaps a dozen times?

Or, as I'm more inclined to believe, did you practice these skills until you felt competent enough in your ability to execute it when needed?

The same should be true about being able to write a PCR.

Now I'm not trying to say one skill is more or less important than the other, it's just some get emphasized more than others.

In EMS we quickly learn to become a "Jack of all trades." A professional able to adjust our game plan on the fly and held accountable for being able to retain a certain level of knowledge while utilizing a varying number of skills depending on the situation we are dealing with.

With every call we respond to, we are responsible for essentially four tasks that must be accomplished with every call:

1. Assess the patient based on their chief complaint, medical history and physical examination.
2. Make an educated differential diagnosis based on our patient assessment.
3. Treat the patient with procedures and transport based on the results of our differential diagnosis.
4. Document the events of the call in a professional and articulate manner that benefits
   a. The Patient
   b. The Provider
   c. The Profession

Each part of our four tasks is dependent on successfully performing the other tasks. Fail to perform one correctly and the other tasks fail as a result.

The PCR ties everything together!

So it is most beneficial to be able to develop and practice the skill of writing strong PCRs

However, after working in EMS for over 20 years, the difference I've noticed between studying a subject such as cardiology or learning a new medical skill like IV placement, as opposed to learning how to write a PCR, is for the majority of us, we start out going into EMT or paramedic school already having a basic ability to write.

Therefore, since the skill of being able to write is not new to us, it often tends to be taken for granted.

However, allow me to paraphrase Jedi Master Qui Gon Jinn, "The ability to *write* does not make you intelligent."

Anyone who writes knows it can be at times a very lonely process, filled with muffled frustrations and just as equally silent successes.

Writing well and with a purpose is a skill that must continuously be practiced and critiqued if one is ever hopeful of getting better at it.

And it's here a lot of people suffer, or stagnate in their PCR skills. If we fail a cardiology exam or are unable to secure an IV out in the field, the feedback is immediate. We can hopefully see what went wrong and fine-tune our study habits or didactic techniques in order to improve and move forward.

But unfortunately after we're done working on our chart and submit it, frequently it disappears into the ether never to be seen or heard from again.

We are regularly left without feedback regarding how affective the details we chose to include in our narrative really were received. Or if the pertinent negatives that we chose to document were helpful in presenting to the reader why the provider did what they did during the course of the call.

The first time I was expected to write an EMS chart was after an interfacility transfer I was called out on. It was my first week working as an EMT cleared by my preceptor (during orientation I wasn't expected to write any PCRs). I remember I tried to write down every single detail I had seen and heard.

This was my usual manner of writing coming from a background in journalism where details are key. For every story I wrote as a journalist, my initial thoughts were to gather as much information and specifics as I could and then put them into words that were clear and accurate.

This was the same approach I took with EMS.

I used my experience being able to condense a scene into words that helped paint an accurate picture in my mind's eye. This was a talent that did not come naturally. I've worked for years learning how to fill a blank page with appropriate words and accurate facts, whether it's a PCR, a magazine article, or a book.

The power of being able to use words effectively was no joke and nothing to be taken lightly.

A healthy respect for the written word has always kept two things in my head when I sit down to write something out. These words I heard from a professor of investigative journalism:

Ambiguity is the Devil's sword

And

Apathy the Devil's shield

Ambiguity is the uncertainty of a message or meaning. Words left unclear are open to any number of interpretations. They have been left unguarded, free to be twisted and manipulated by someone more skilled at using words than you are into something you never intended or meant to say.

It's a deceptive skill more powerful than Thor's hammer. The Devil's sword is often wielded by attorneys looking to find discrepancies, inconsistencies, or ill-chosen words that might aid their clients' version of events.

Apathy is the indifference or lack of concern people might feel towards a particular thing. It's the perfect shield for complacency, mediocracy and injustice to breed. It's exactly what Irish philosopher; Edmund Burke meant when he said, "*All evil needs is for good men to do nothing.*" Burke realized that a lot of injustice and malpractice can occur in plain sight if nobody cares to look.

Which is why I decided to write this book!

This book is intended for the first responder who is familiar with the rudimentary processes of how to conduct a patient assessment and knowledgeable of the basic legal terms taught in an EMS course.

I'm hopeful this book will help to clarify any aspects of EMS reporting that might be confusing or unclear. To bolster confidence in the words you choose to write down on paper. And, to help you see just how much your report can make an impactful difference, not just for your patient, but also, for your profession and for yourself.

I want to take some of the anxiety out of what should and should not go into writing a report, as well as take away some of the ambiguity that comes with the reasons why it is so important.

I've intentionally written this book so that the chapters will be brief! They're short enough so they can be read quickly and labeled so they can be easily referenced while out in the field.

I have included a review of the three most common formats of EMS reports in use today: SOAP-E, CHART-E and a straight narrative. Each is detailed, with specifics noting the variations in each and a breakdown of how to best organize each one.

Several of the chapters in this book address certain legal specifics that in the event you are ever called into court to defend what you've written hopefully will help keep you from sinking into litigious quicksand.

The importance of being able to have your PCRs critiqued is covered, including who you might be able to ask for quicker feedback and constructive interventions.

And finally a large portion of this book will be spent dealing with specific calls you might go on along with the many details and questions you might want to ask and document. At the end of each chapter a sample chart is included for reference and to help serve as a template for your own PCRs,

Unfortunately what this book, or any other book for that matter, won't do is instantaneously give you the ability to write a PCR well. That will come with time, practice and constructive criticism.

Equally unfortunate is the fact that often times you can work your entire career in EMS writing subpar or maybe "just barely adequate to get by" charts and nobody will call you on it.

Writing stronger EMS charts is something that

you are going to have to **want** to do!

It has to be an intrinsic desire of pride, integrity and a matter of dedication that will drive a person to devote themselves to working on this aspect of their career.

Because much like the charts you write, the benefits might not be immediately seen.

This book should elevate your awareness of how important what you document really is and how it plays into the overall matrix of patient care, funding for your department or service, an elevation of training standards and patient care, and serve as the basis for future research and development to help continue to push EMS standards into the 21st century.

I also, hopefully will get you to appreciate the sheer power and impact of the written word.

The first part of this book is divided into 10 chapters that will give you not just a proper foundation for being able to write and produce a stronger patient care report, but also an understanding and appreciation for why it is so important to develop these skills.

You will see that what you write affects not just you or your patient, but also the profession as a whole!

The second and third parts of this book are divided into various medical and trauma calls you might respond to. Each chapter will provide you with several questions that might be important to ask and details you will be important for you to document.

Once you are done reading this book hopefully you will see that the ability to write a strong PCR gives you the ability to level the playing field. The blank page doesn't care if you're a chief or a rookie, a paramedic or EMT, doctor or nurse. The content you choose to include or omit will be entirely dependent on you.

Words you choose to use can either paint a realistic picture of what you saw, or serve to confuse and mislead someone away from what you intended. So great care and proper respect should be given to each word you choose to use.

For as the playwright Eric Bogosian once wrote, *"Sticks and stones can break bones, but words cause permanent damage."*

Chapter 1

What Is a Patient Care Report?

Depending on where you work and how many years you decide to invest in this profession, chances are pretty reasonable you will respond to hundreds, if not thousands of EMS calls throughout the course of your career. Each call you respond to, every patient contact you encounter, every refusal you take and every false alarm you respond to will have their own unique story. And each story will require a detailed report that you will be required to write and stand behind.

But the question still remains...

What is a PCR?

Once it's been written and submitted, where does it go? Who reads it? And what overall part does your PCR play in benefiting:

1. **Your Patient**
2. **You the Provider**
3. **And the Profession as a whole**

I call these the three priority "Ps" of PCR documentation.

And the answer to all of them is the same:

"It depends."

It depends on how well you are able to address the various needs each of these priorities requires to be answered.

Once written, your PCR becomes many things to so many different people:

- To some, such as ER physicians or nurses, it can become an immediate piece of vital information used in the continuation of patient care.
- To others, it becomes a necessary document used for billing, which helps to generate funds for your department or service. This is money generated that goes into paying your salary, purchasing new supplies and used to buy new equipment or maintain existing resources.
- It's used also used by Quality Assurance to ensure for the overall standard of care is consistently being met. Your PCR can be used to help develop new protocols, or develop new research in order to broaden the horizons of EMS as a profession.
- Your training department might use your PCR as a lesson plan to emphasize an example of quality care, or to correct a problem so that you and your colleagues can avoid repeating the same mistake.

- If your patient happened to be deceased, law enforcement, the medical examiner or coroner might read your report to look for what details you chose to document. Many times they are looking for any possible details or discrepancies that might aid in their own investigation of trying to piece together what might have happened.
- And finally, but certainly not least of which, it's a CYA legal defense against possible lawsuits. The strongest defense a first responder has against successfully being sued or being held negligent and liable is to follow your standard of care and to show this by carefully, systematically and methodically documenting all the events and actions which occurred during the course of the 911 call.

Same report, but looked at for so many different reasons.

For now we'll focus on the priority three "Ps" of PCR reporting: Patient, Provider, and Profession. Many of what you will find listed here are covered in depth later on in their own individual chapters, but I still wanted to list most of what I look for in my standard PCR.

A patient care report is a single point of view, written usually by the first responder in charge of patient care, detailing how the EMS responder perceived the events of what occurred throughout the course of an EMS call. And while there are many different narrative and charting formats (some of which we'll cover in detail later in this book) many of the details that you should be thinking about and documenting are the same for every report.

The report should be a clear and accurate detailing of:

- Time EMS crew was dispatched, for what reason and in what manner they responded (non-emergent or lights and sirens)
- Time of arrival to scene, including any exceptions, such as traffic delays, or staging for scene safety
- Patient position upon your arrival (patient found lying prone on the ground loudly crying, patient found walking around in the front yard clutching his chest, patient found lying supine, unconscious, unresponsive, no pulse, not breathing)
- Any suspicious or unusual scene conditions (several empty bottles of alcohol found near patient, heavy amounts of trash or clutter found in front room impeding EMS extraction of patient, multiple piles of animal feces smeared into carpet and walls presenting an overall unhealthy atmosphere to perform patient assessment on scene)
- Patient assessment:

Clues and details of what to look for during specific medical, trauma and environmental calls covered later in book.

- Vital signs (should be at least two, but more is better if we are going to trend patient condition over the course of our call)
- Time of departure to hospital
- Your diagnostic diagnosis (very important for so many reasons including your justification for interventions, packaging and transport decisions, as well as ICD-10 codes for billing)
- A full list of treatments that you decide to provide (including time, dose and route your interventions were given)
- Document number of attempts and successes for any intervention you perform (IV access attempted, twice unsuccessfully in patient's right hand, successful insertion in left A/C with Normal Saline at a rate of TKO: this gives your training and Quality Assurance valuable information on what may need to be covered in future trainings, product deficiencies, department statistics in performance of certain skills. Never be afraid to document unsuccessful attempts. This might just be something like a technique or some other matter that needs to be looked at and corrected in order for YOU to become a better provider and for your patients to receive the best treatment)
- Any pertinent negatives (covered later in the book)

- A full set of demographics: name, address, phone number, social security number, insurance information
- If the patient could not speak English and required a translator: who provided it
- If you needed to contact Medical Control: a brief reason why you had to call, the name of the physician and if possible, verbatim retelling of what their orders were
- How patient responds to your treatments (better or worse?)
- Time of arrival at hospital
- Mileage from scene to hospital (if your ambulance doesn't have a way to automatically track this, you may have to 'zero' out your odometer prior to transport)
- A PATIENT SIGNATURE (Very Important! Most services cannot bill insurance without it.)
- If the Patient is Unable To Sign: document exactly why they are unable to. Do not just put PUTS, this is a vague term that most insurance companies will reject. (document exactly why the patient could not sign: patient unable to sign due to altered mentation exhibited secondary to head trauma incurred from MVC, patient unable to sign due inability to move hands secondary to current complaint of paralysis from neck down, patient unable to sign secondary to being unconscious)

- Reason for need for transport by ambulance: perhaps just as important as a signature is documenting why the patient required transport by ambulance. (Do not simply put Patient Confined to Bed or Patient Unable to Ambulate as reasons. Again these are vague terms that should be explained in more detail: patient confined to bed due to chronic paralysis of both legs, patient unable to ambulate due to morbid obesity resulting in inability to bear weight on legs, patient required ambulance transport due to need for albuterol nebulized treatment due to shortness of breath and wheezing secondary to chronic asthma)
- The name and title of the person you turned over patient care to.
- Any other exceptions you think may need to be included (closest hospital, Eastside, was on divert, transport destination changed to: Northside Hospital, upon arrival at hospital, remained on scene for 30 minutes waiting for room assignment)

Whew! That's an awfully long grocery list of information that should be included into one EMS report.

However you can see that by including all of this information it takes into consideration and addresses information needed to satisfy each of your priority three "Ps" (Patient, Provider, Profession).

There's something included that keeps each of these vested interests satisfied.

The hospital will be interested in how the patient was found, their chief complaint and what you did on scene and en route to the hospital.

The provider will be able to cover their behind in the event this ever goes to court as it thoroughly demonstrates and documents quality patient care DID NOT stray from the standard of care expected from someone with your level of training.

The profession will look for billing information, QA parameters and training opportunities.

However it all starts with you!

Unlike the actual running of an EMS call which involves teamwork, coordination and cooperation, writing a PCR is not a collaborative process.

It's one author documenting one point of view. At times there may be cause to have more than one medical provider documenting and submitting a PCR on the same patient, however this usually involves the transfer of care from one responder to another.

i.e. Paramedic Jones from Fire Department X is first on scene and begins initial patient care, which includes a primary survey and baseline set of vital signs.

Paramedic Smith from Ambulance Service Y, which has the transport contract for the county, arrives on scene. Jones briefs Smith on the patient's chief complaint and condition and helps to load the patient up into the back of Smith's ambulance. Smith assumes patient care and transports the patient into the hospital. Both medical responders will have PCRs written on the same patient: however there is no guarantee these reports do not contradict each other or even remotely sound like they are treating the same patient. What they should have however, is a clear, accurate representation of what each provider saw, were told, and what they did.

To help you, I would suggest documenting your findings as you uncover them. Take notes… a lot of notes throughout the call. I used to write on my gloves all the time. However I also lost a lot of my notes as I would frequently change gloves, either because I needed to assess more than one patient or I got blood or some other biohazard on my gloves requiring a change.

Oops… there went my notes.

I now carry a small blank notebook, the type you typically see reporters at news conferences carry. I scribble notes on it, things my patient might say, details about the scene, vital signs, medication lists etc. If I forgot, or don't have a notebook, I will often tear off a 6" length strip of 1" white tape and put it on my thigh and "presto chango" I have a place to write notes.

Be careful though!

The thing you have to remember about taking such copious amounts of notes on something other than your PCR is where your notes eventually end up. Don't just throw them away in the trash as they often have patient information on them that can be a HIPAA violation.

While the majority of PCRs are now being typed into a Toughbook computer, it is not uncommon for first responders to be required to write out on an initial report on an actual paper form in order to leave something tangible with the ER staff.

However once your PCR is written out and submitted, it instantly becomes a restricted document, limited for viewing by only those who have either direct care of your patient (doctors, nurses), responsible for supervision or training of the provider (QA, Training/Educators, Direct Supervisors), those responsible for billing, those conducting a legal investigation into a crime, and those authorized by the patient to access or subpoena their medical records.

Point is, not everyone can just look at your PCR. It is a secure document containing very personal and very private patient information. You are given a tremendous amount of trust by the public at large to come into their home on perhaps the worst night of their lives and asked to take care of someone. Please do not ever violate that sacred trust by doing something stupid like posting information on Facebook, or gossiping about your patient with another provider. The information you acquire is part of the trust that patient extends to you.

It's nobody else's business.

And one final word on procrastination. As Charles Dickens has said, "*It is the thief of time.*" Do not fall into the trap of trying to put off documentation until a later time. Your patient deserves better.

You would never hold off administering Nitro to a patient with chest pain until later, or hold off on oxygen for someone with dyspnea until you better rested. The same standard should be held for your PCR.

You have the strongest recollection of what went on during the call just after you turn patient care over to someone else.

But make no mistake, the instant your call is over, your memory of the images, details and incidents begins to fade at a startlingly rapid rate. And while your notes will certainly help to fill in finer details, it's your unique memory of what happened that will really be the paint from which you will begin to color your picture.

If you put off writing your chart until later, because of food, fatigue or friends draw you away from your responsibilities; you may quickly find you have two… maybe three, or even more charts to write at the end of your shift. Suddenly, you are now forced to try and recall specific information from a number of events that occurred sometimes hours ago.

It's a poor habit to get into and a tremendous disservice to your patient, your profession and yourself.

One thing you can do to help yourself is learn how to write your PCRs quicker with less hesitation of how to begin or what information to include or not include. This comes with repetition and practice. However, we do utilize certain PCR formats that help to organize our information making it faster to document and submit.

So let's take a look at a few of the more common types of PCR formats we use in EMS and the specifics that go with each one of them.

And remember, the way I am detailing how to document your information into a PCR is simply the way I find it to be the quickest, easiest and most effective way of doing it. Of course you are going to develop your own style and that's ok.

After all, 5 + 5 will always equal 10, but so does 6 + 4, 7 + 3 etc... The point is there are several ways to get to the same correct answer. So read on and see if the way I choose to write strong EMS reports is for you or if you'd prefer to tweak it a bit to fit your style. In any case...

I'll see you, in Chapter 2!

Chapter 2

CHART-E

CHART-E along with SOAP-E are two of the most commonly used acronyms in EMS reporting. Each format helps to breakdown massive amounts of information that a first responder might retrieve during an EMS call so it can be organized into a logical, easy to understand format.

This is extremely important for documentation!

Your PCR will be skimmed by some searching only for specific tidbits of information, while others will scrutinize your report looking for what you decided to include and not include into your legal document.

So knowing how to use acronyms such as CHART-E becomes an extremely effective way to document the information you want to present.

The trick to using acronyms is to understand what piece of information goes where. Each letter of an acronym used for EMS reporting represents an expectation of information that should provide the reader a quick way to reference what they are looking for.

In EMS **CHART-E** commonly stands for:

- **C: Chief Complaint**
- **H: History**

- **A: Assessment**
- **Rx: Treatment**
- **T: Transport**
- **E: Exceptions**

Think of each of these letters as a skeleton and the information we provide as the organs, muscles and tissue we are going to use to eventually build a person.

Each letter represents a bullet point of information that we are going to be expected to fully flesh out and answer.

Since we are writing for several different audiences, we have to constantly be thinking about what each of them want to know and what they are going to be expecting in each portion of your PCR.

Lucky for us, if we are just simply aware of these expectations, it becomes infinitely easier to include them without QA or billing having to send it back to you for corrections and addendums.

So where do we begin?

As with all good stories... we start at the beginning.

C: Chief Complaint- I usually start out with how and why I was dispatched followed by a timestamp of when I arrived on scene.

This starts your internal narrative.

Once I arrive on scene I will note any odd or unusual details that help to paint a picture of how I interpret the scene. This is followed by a quick set of demographics to frame the context of who my patient is and then a brief statement of what their chief complaint is. If you're able to utilize the patient's own words to notate what their chief complaint is this is often an effective descriptive way to note this.

Remember if you choose to use your patient's exact words, use quotation marks and document them exactly as your patient said them.

- *Medic 51 dispatched Code 3 for male patient shortness of breath. Upon arrival (1917) heavy odor of cigarette smoke along with numerous ashtrays overflowing with cigarette butts noted in front room where Pt is a 48 y/o male found sitting upright in tripod position c/o "I can't breathe!"*
- *Rescue 2 dispatched Code 3 for female complaining of abdominal pain. Upon arrival (0902) Pt is a 58 y/o female found lying supine on the ground, guarding her abdomen with knees flexed to her chest, c/o extreme LLQ abdominal pain.)*

A physician typically is not going to be interested in how you were dispatched or how you responded. That's usually just more words that they have to slog through in order to get to the meat of what his patient's main problem are that brought him to the hospital by ambulance.

So keep it brief!

H: History- This section of CHART-E is basically used to document what has happened to our patient prior to him calling 911. We're interested in how long our patient has been suffering with whatever caused him to activate 911, how he's been treating it and how well that self-treatment has been going. We're interested in any co-morbidities that might be affecting the chief complaint, what medications he's on and if he's been compliant with them, and what general lifestyle our patient has. So to this end I recommend that you break down this section into three different parts: hpi (history of present illness), pmh (past medical history) and s/lsh (social/lifestyle history).

- **hpi**: Typically if the problem is medical in nature I follow the **OPQRST** mnemonic to document my history of present illness:
  -**Onset** (*What were you doing when pain started?*)
  -**Provocation/Palliation** (*Does anything make it better or worse?*)
  -**Quality** (*Can you describe the pain?*)
  -**Radiation** (*Where does the pain originate and does it radiate anywhere?*)
  -**Severity** (*On a scale from 1 to 10, how bad does your pain feel?*)

-Time of onset (*How long have you been suffering with this problem and have you done anything to help treat it?*)

(At 0740 *pt states he was asleep in bed when pain woke him. Pain increases when pt lies supine and engages in exercise, and decreases with rest in a seated position. Pt describes pain as "crushing" pain which is constant and unyielding. Pain originates in the substernal region and radiates into left shoulder and down left arm. Pt rates pain a 10/10 in severity and states pt has been suffering with chest pain for 3 days, slowly increasing in severity until this morning when pain became unbearable it reached this level of discomfort 20 minutes prior to EMS activation. Pt states that he has been self-medicating with alcohol, specifically vodka, which patient states he's been increasing the amount he consumes to match his elevation of pain discomfort.*)
If the problem is traumatic in nature without a medical component i.e. a motor vehicle crash (MVC) I will have documented the complaint and problem under C: Chief Complaint section and will only need to use the H: History section for past medical history (pmh).

- **pmh**: To obtain a quick medical history I use the **SAMPLE** acronym:
  -Signs and Symptoms (*Remember we "see" signs, a patient tells us their symptoms.*)

-**Allergies** (*Is patient allergic to any medications?*)

-**Medications:** (use the acronym **PORCH** for medications)

    -**Prescribed** (*Includes meds they are not taking but doctor has prescribed.*)

    -**Over the Counter** (*Why are they taking these OTC meds?*)

    -**Recreational** (*Illicit or otherwise*)

    -**Compliant** (*Is patient compliant with taking their medications?*)

    -**Herbs and Supplements** – (*Is there anything that might be of note?*)

-**Past Medical History**: (*This should match up, at least in part, with the medications that you listed. If you've got Glucophage listed as a medication, chances are this patient has a medical history of Diabetes, regardless of they say so or not. Often I've found patients who are able to maintain chronic problems, like blood pressure or diabetes, no longer consider them a medical problem so they neglect to list it when asked. That will be something you will have to clarify!*)

-**Events Leading Up to Present Illness:** (*This will have typically already been answered in your **OPQRST**, but if it's a traumatic call you may have to ask this.*)

- **s/lsh**: Use the acronym **SASS** to find out about a patient's social and lifestyle history.

-Sedentary: (*Does the patient appear to be obese, emaciated, frail or weak? A question about physical activity and if they are they able to walk without getting immediately exhausted, short of breath, is important to know.*)

-Alcohol: (*Does the patient consume alcohol on a regular basis? How much do they consume? Have they ever gone into withdrawals without alcohol?*)

- Sexual activity: (*If this is a female with abdominal pain, a question about if they are sexually active is very appropriate.*)

-Smoker: (*Does the patient smoke cigarettes or cigars? How much do they smoke in a day? How long have they been smoking?*)

A: Assessment- This is your ability to include what you found during your initial assessment. These should be your **objective** findings. If the patient is a trauma patient you're probably going to want to include a full head to toe assessment.

Remember anything you do not include in your report: DID NOT HAPPEN! So don't skip.

Use the DCAP-BTLS acronym to help you when searching for obvious and occult injuries. (*Deformities, Crepitus/Contusions, Abrasions, Punctures, Burns, Tenderness, Lacerations, Swelling*) This should be done if your patient has been involved in a traumatic accident, unconscious, or presenting with an altered mentation. We need to rule out possible reasons for the unconsciousness or altered mentation.

You can choose to write your assessment from head-to-toe. I have seen very nicely written reports that include a list of body systems and their assessment of each. Regardless of how you choose to document your physical assessment, do one and be thorough.

If your patient's main complaint is medical in nature: i.e. chest pain or shortness of breath. Some form of physical assessment must be documented. A good rule of thumb I use for physically assessing a medical patient is to examine the:

EYES, NECK, CHEST, ABDOMEN and EXTREMITIES: this gives you a fast overview of the overall physical presentation of your patient. If something leads to a more thorough examination of a particular part of the body or closer scrutiny of a body system, then by all means be like Christopher Columbus and explore and explore some more!

- Eyes: I'm looking to see if they are PERL (Pupils are Equal Round and Reactive To Light) Are they unusually pinpoint as in an opioid overdose, or overly dilated which may be indicative of a stimulant problem.
- Neck: Look to see if there are any signs of Jugular Venous Distention, Tracheal Deviation, and

palpate the posterior for any traumatic deformities or step-offs.

- Chest: Symmetrical rise and fall of the chest with each respiration. Palpate for any instabilities, have patient try to take a deep breath with your hands on their rib cage, feeling for any crepitus, and asking if patient has any pain upon deep respiration. Listen to lung sounds auscultating for adventitious sounds.
- Extremities: Palpate each extremity feeling for DCAP-BTLS. Be sure to note if something is present on one side or bilateral. Check each extremity for PMS (*Pulse Motor Sensory*) and inspect for any signs of edema, especially in lower extremities. If present, note the pitting length (+1. +2, etc) and note how far up edema extends. (*Pitting edema noted bilateral feet present up to mid-calf region of lower leg.*)

An assessment of patient's mental status and affect should be noted, especially if it appears to be outside of obvious normal parameters or is found to be a pertinent negative.

REMEMBER YOU NEED TO DETERMINE IF THIS IS A CHRONIC PROBLEM OR AN ACUTE SITUATION!!!

For instance: If you have a patient who is elderly and presenting with signs of dementia do not assume this is a chronic state for this patient. Look for family, friends and medications as a possible lead to answer the Chronic vs. Acute question. If none are available, I recommend a thorough head to toe physical exam looking for clues, such as signs of trauma to help solve this mystery. ALWAYS ERR ON THE SIDE OF CAUTION; IF YOU CAN GET NO INFORMATION, THIS IS ACUTE UNTIL PROVEN OTHERWISE.

Your assessment should end with a clearly defined differential diagnosis. This is the bridge that will carry you over to the Rx portion of your chart. How you choose to proceed with your field treatment should be based on what your perceived diagnosis is.

EXAMPLE: *ddx: chest pain secondary to possible MI.*

Rx: Treatment- Your treatment should include every intervention you provided on scene. There should be a clear, logical thread from your stated differential diagnosis (ddx) detailed in the assessment section that supports each one of your interventions.

For example, if your ddx was chest pain, you should have interventions that follow your standard of care:

> EMT: Oxygen @ (1733)
>
> Aspirin @ (1736)
>
> Assist patient with their own Nitro @ (1739)

Paramedic:

Intravenous Access @ (1742)

ECG   @ (1743)

12-Lead @ (1744)

Analgesic if needed @ (1750)

Each one of your interventions should have a timestamp on it to allow for an easy to follow timeline. (*ex. asa 324mg PO @ 1533, o2 therapy started 4 lpm via N/C @ 2100*) Vital signs after your treatment therapy has been initiated should be included here with a timestamp to allow for clear trending of your patient's progress or regress.

One phrase you should utilize when wrapping up your Treatment section is:

Pt required ambulance transport due to...

Simply stating why this patient has to go into the hospital by ambulance will help your PCR with billing and eventually being reimbursed by insurance companies. Remember, there are all sorts of reasons why a patient needs to go into the hospital by ambulance! If your patient has any complaint, injury or possible ailments that would raise a cause for you to think they need transport by ambulance, **STATE IT!**

(*Pt required ambulance transport due to being unable to ambulate on their own without risk of harm due to complaint of dizziness and shortness of breath. Pt required ambulance transport due to need for continuous oxygen administration which they do not have on their own. Pt required ambulance transport due to morbid obesity making it impossible for them to bear weight on their own and fit inside their own personal vehicle. Pt required ambulance transport due to stated suicidal ideology, making him a possible threat to himself.*)

You also should support your assumption by stating on your chart the care you provided in getting your patient from the point you found them to the point where they got on your gurney. Hopefully, you will be limiting (ideally eliminating) the need for patient to move to the gurney on their own, instead you and your crew took the time and put in the effort to move the patient to your gurney.

This helps to eliminate the possibility your patient might fall while under your care. It also substantiates the need for your patient to require transport by ambulance.

Even if your patient is ambulatory, you can still state that the patient requires ambulance transport due to any number of reasons. It is a rare patient who absolutely has no real reason to go to the hospital. And even then, if your patient is a 911 system abuser, I would argue that this patient is crying out for help and may need ambulance transport for possible psychological issues.

T: Transport- Once the patient has been placed onto the gurney- document your destination and in what manner you are running to the hospital- *hot or cold*. You will need to provide a full reassessment of the treatments you initiated on scene to follow through with how the patient responded to them (*did they get better or are they still getting worse?*)

You might also list new interventions that you may not have time to address while on scene, i.e. secondary injuries, splining, etc. Again each of these interventions should include a timestamp on it to underscore a linear timeline from the moment you first got on scene until the time you turned your patient over to the hospital.

You will also want to include a mention you sent a radio report to the hospital advising them of what you're bringing and if they had a bed assigned for you or if you're heading to Triage.

A secondary assessment focused on a slower more methodical head to toe physical exam is customarily performed in the ambulance heading back to the hospital.

Note anything of importance you may not have addressed or noticed during your primary assessment.

If you are turning your patient care over to another ground or air ambulance, include the reason why (*i.e. traffic and long distance so patient turned over to helicopter crew*), who you turned your patient over to and when.

E: Exceptions- Exceptions are basically anything that occurred during the course of the call that was unusual or out of the ordinary. Examples of this would include:

- Difficulty arriving on scene due to traffic
- Sent to wrong address
- Prolonged extrication due to patient entrapment
- Delay getting to patient due to scene safety issues
- Remained on scene to help patient find her glasses
- Left patient's pet with a neighbor

Through sheer repetition you should gain enough speed to produce a PCRs that's fast, clear and accurate. However your goal should be more. You want strong, detailed PCR's that provide enough information to satisfy all who are going to read it.

You could easily include enough details in the CHART-E so you wouldn't need to include a separate narrative, but I believe that is a mistake, especially if you are just starting out. It takes time and experience to remember all the details required to put into a CHART-E, and you want to keep your PCR streamlined so it doesn't look cluttered with information that may not be needed.

Breaking up long paragraphs into smaller bites is also recommended. Otherwise, your PCR becomes an exercise in patience and scrutiny as the reader tries to wade through endless details searching for specific information they are looking for.

Another tip that I cannot stress more highly is to avoid procrastination like the plague! As soon as you turn your patient over, try to resist the temptation to take a break, eat or fall asleep.

Details fade quickly!

The longer you wait to write your report, the more prone it is to have information jumbled or details forgotten. Throughout my career, I tried my best to avoid procrastination when it came to writing my reports. I knew that if I put it off until "later" my documentation wouldn't be as strong or as detailed as it could be. Also, there wasn't anything worse than getting close to the end of a long, busy shift and having to face a pile of half written reports I needed to complete before I could leave.

The CHART-E method of taking notes is how I initially learned how to write PCRs by hand in Albuquerque, New Mexico working for Albuquerque Ambulance Service (AAS). We were an extremely busy system that seemed to always be on the go!

I loved it!

I loved the fast pace each shift presenting me with. Every day I went into my job not knowing what I might face or what challenges I would be asked to overcome. And along with working so many shifts and responding to so many calls, AAS also provided me with an ample opportunity to learn how to practice write a complete and thorough CHART-E.

Now I'm not going to lie to you, knowing how to type helped me immensely. Working for years a spell in journalism taught me how to type fast with a fair amount of accuracy. I would highly recommend to anyone who is in EMS and has to "peck" at their keyboard, to do themselves a favor and take a typing course to increase your speed. Ten years from now, you'll thank me for this advice!

Here is an example of what I would consider a complete CHART-E of a traumatic incident. The details presented are written in a way that are easy to find and completes a fluid timeline from arrival to turning over patient to the hospital. It also address the issue of need for ambulance transport.

CHART- E example:

C: Medic 51 responded code 3 for reported two vehicle MVA (1719). Arrival on scene (1723) positioning ambulance in front of responding Engine. No gas spills noted on ground or other obvious scene safety concerns. Police units on scene to divert traffic around scene. Traffic safety vests donned by ambulance crew in addition to standard PPE.

Upon our arrival Pt is a 27 y/o female found awake and tracking EMS upon approach, c/o neck and back pain. Pt states, "My neck is hurting me so much!" Pt found in the driver's seat of a mid-sized automobile, Chevy Equinox (black) which was struck on the driver's side by an SUV, Chevy Traverse (grey), causing approximately 10" of intrusion into driver's compartment. Pt states that she was restrained with shoulder and lap belt at time of accident, but unsecured herself after the initial collision. Pt denies loss of consciousness (LOC) and states she remembers the events of the MVC without difficulty.

H: hpi: Pt was stopped at a stop light at the intersection of Lomas Blvd and Central Ave when according to patient, the light turned green, she went out into intersection and was struck by an SUV going through a red light. The approximate time of the accident was 1715, the weather at time of collision was clear and sunny.

   pmh: Pt has a past medical history of anxiety and bi-polar disorder. She takes risperidon and St.

John's wart and has been compliant with her medications according to the prescription written by her doctor. She denies any medical allergies. She denies being a smoker of tobacco, but does occasionally use medical marijuana from time to time that is not prescribed to her. She describes herself as a social drinker consuming only a drink or two every month.

A: Pt found awake and oriented to situation sitting upright in the driver's side of her vehicle holding her neck. The seatbelt at time of EMS arrival was not secured. Airbag deployment from steering wheel, starred windshield. Pt has no obvious immediate life threats that are noted. Pt able to speak in multi-word sentences without difficulty. Pt denies any shortness of breath, but does appear anxious and upset. Pt skin warm, pink and dry. Pulse strong and regular at the radial. Pt advised to stay still and not move her head. C-spine precautions taken (1725). Small lacerations noted on patient's forehead, and hands, lots of broken glass around patient from shattered driver's side window. Driver's side door pried open by hand and backboard placed on driver's side.

Pt rotated by EMS and Fire crews so her head is lowered onto the backboard and her pelvis, and legs slid up the backboard and onto a gurney. (1729)

Prior to strapping patient to backboard, she was covered with a sheet and her clothes were cut off to expose for any occult injuries.

Rapid head to toe assessment noted no deformities in head, face or skull only slight lacerations previously noted. Neck palpated with tenderness in cervical region, no step-offs or deformities noted. No signs of tracheal deviation or JVD. Chest presents with equal rise and fall with each respiration. No deformities or crepitus noted in intercostal or sternal regions. Slight tenderness upon palpation of left side. Abdominal region presented with slight distention and rigidity on left upper quadrant. Three other quadrants palpated and found to be unremarkable. Pelvis is stable without pain or tenderness. Lower extremities present without injury: good bilateral PMS without incident. Upper extremities present with slight lacerations on both hands and forearms. No other injuries noted. Bilateral PMS is good and presents without incident. Pt logrolled to right side and her posterior was visualized and palpated. No signs of deformity contusions or abrasions noted from occiput of skull, down through cervical, thoracic and lumbar spine. Pt secured to backboard in full spinal immobilization. (1731) no change in extremity PMS S/P immobilization.

Pt required ambulance transport due to significant mechanism of injury which could result in further injury from possible spinal cord or internal hemorrhage if left to go by any other means. DDX: possible multi-system trauma including spinal cord injury and internal hemorrhage.

R: Code 3 to UNMH (1734), Medic Serino and EMT Rogers in back attending to patient. Pt remained awake and very talkative throughout transport. Baseline vitals (1735): P: 108, R: 20 equal and regular, B/P 132/78, Pulse Ox 94% Room air-Serino.

Supplemental oxygen started 4 lpm via N/C (1737). IV access 16g L A/C, initiated at (1740), IV ran at TKO.

V/S (1740): P: 112, R 22, B/P 128/74 Pulse Ox 97% on 4 lpm via N/C- Rogers.

ECG shows Sinus Tach without ectopy or ST elevation (1743). 12-Lead ECG is unremarkable for ST elevation (1748). Secondary assessment performed. Lacerations bandaged by EMT Rogers. Abdomen on LUQ appears slightly more distended and patient is complaining that her abdomen hurts. Pt rates pain a 10/10 indicating that the pain does not radiate anywhere. She is also complaining of neck pain rated an 8/10 and a headache rated a 6/10 in severity.

V/S (1750): P 110, R 20, B/P 124/62 Pulse Ox 98% on 4 lpm via N/C- Rogers

Radio report made to UNMH by Serino (17:50) advising ER staff of patient condition and ETA.

V/S (1755): P 104, R 18, B/P 108/58, Pulse Ox 98 % 4 lpm via N/C, Capnography 42- Serino

Arrival at hospital (1758). No change in patient's mentation or complaints. Pt turned over to ER RN Stacy Wheeler who put patient in Room 1. Report made to ER staff including Dr. Forrester who assumed patient care.

E: Delay getting to patient due to heavy traffic and poor routing by computer navigated system which directed EMS down an avenue with heavy construction.

Chapter 3

SOAP-E

SOAP-E is one of the most common acronyms found in EMS reporting. It is divided up into basically 4 main sections:

- What you're told.   (S: subjective)
- What you see.   (O: objective)
- What you assessed   (A: assessment)
- And, what you did.   (P: plan)
- E is for Exceptions: same as found in CHART-E

I love the SOAP-E format as I find it almost the perfect blend of the CHART-E format and a simple freeform narrative format. It allows for a looser style of writing that can be easier and faster to produce than writing a CHART-E. However there are more expectations that have to be met in each section of SOAP-E if you hope to keep your PCR appearing professional and effective.

Certain portions of this chapter will be very similar to what was written in the previous chapter and in the spirit of trying to eliminate redundancy as much as possible, you may be directed back to Chapter 2 at certain points during this chapter.

When someone looks at a PCR written in SOAP-E, they are expecting specific information to be found in certain sections: and when they're not, things can get missed.

For example, if you were writing a PCR in the CHART-E format, you wouldn't expect to find information about what you did en route to the hospital in the history portion of the chart.

It just simply doesn't belong there.

Our PCR's should never turn into a tedious game of "hide and seek" for specific information as time is often a factor when someone is scanning your chart.

So in order to keep our PCR on the side that is helpful rather than the alternative, it helps to know what goes where.

And, silly as this might seem, but the more letters you decide to use for an acronym, the less information you usually have to include in each section. Each letter divides up and evenly distributes the information in an organized, agreed upon manner. CHART-E has one more letter than SOAP-E, so it can be broken down into smaller blocks.

S: Subjective- This is the information that your patient tells you. From the moment you arrive on scene, you should be on high alert noting details and gathering information. Listen to what your patient is telling you;

both verbally and non-verbally! Information is relayed in many different ways.

The S: subjective section is your chance to detail relevant information based on what you are taking in with the three senses we normally use in EMS: visual, touch and smell.

- Note the time of your arrival
- If you arrive on scene and the patient's house is cluttered with empty pizza boxes and there is rodent feces on the ground: your patient is telling you something!
- If you find empty pill bottles thrown around the apartment: your patient is telling you something!
- Or if you see a gun lying on the ground: your patient is telling you something!

These are all examples of information that you are taking in, but haven't been actually told by your patient. Your S: subjective section should start with your arrival on scene and a timestamp so you can begin the fluid timeline that proceeds throughout the EMS call finishing when you timestamp the moment of patient transfer of care to the hospital staff.

You should provide a general impression of what you are seeing as you approach your patient.

- Note the gender of your patient
- Their approximate age and weight

- Their activity and position as you approach (*for example are they tracking you or not tracking you, are they ambulatory without assistance pacing around the room or are they laying supine, crying out in pain*)

Note if this is your only patient or if he is 1 of 2 or 3 etc...

What is your patient's chief complaint?

- If possible use your patient's own words if they help to illustrate the severity of the situation or possibly used as a pertinent negative. Remember to use quotation marks if you are directly quoting your patient and making sure to attribute who referenced the quote.

What is your patient's history?

- hpi: We would include the full OPQRST if the problem is medical. If it's a traumatic injury a detailed event of what happened.
- pmh: Get a full detailed SAMPLE history from your patient. Remember, a medical emergency can precede a traumatic event, so be on the lookout for possible medical causes to traumatic injuries.

This section is basically written by what you see and what you are told by your patient. You need to be certain that you do not in any way interject your own personal opinions or assumptions into this section.

Use the words "possibly," or "the appearance of," if you are trying to pinpoint something that walks like a duck, talks like a duck, but you do not know for sure if it's actually a duck. The bird has the appearance of a duck. The bird possibly is a duck due to the observed webbed feet, quacks and swims on the top of the water.

This allows you to not be pinned down by a lawyer later on who might say, "*Mr. Serino, are you an expert in ornithology? Are you an expert in identification of the bird family anatidae?*"

- To both questions I would have to say, "*No.*"

"*But Mr. Serino in your medical chart you make reference to your patient as being a duck. How can you be so certain with your limited, to zero expertise in this field?*"

"*Uh oh, game over.*"

Now the same situation could be applied to a more medical scenario, such as if a first responder makes the mistake of saying, "*The patient was drunk.*"

"*Mr. Serino are you an expert in the limits of what constitutes intoxication?*" And the lawyer tears my chart to pieces.

It's much better to stay noncommittal. State your point, but don't ever get pinned down by it unless you can substantiate it.

- *If a patient appears intoxicated from alcohol, state patient had the appearance of possible intoxication due to staggered gait, bloodshot eyes, odor of alcohol coming of the patient, and the number of empty gin bottles littered on the floor that the patient admits to consuming tonight.*

O: Objective- in this section you are expected to document what you see. This could be also seen as signs that you observe, whereas symptoms would be in the first section.

These signs could be obvious observations: *(Pt presenting with left hand clutching his chest in a Levine's sign. Pt appears diaphoretic and pale. Pt speaking in one to two word sentences with obvious adventitious lung sounds noted.)*

This is also a spot where you can write down obvious pertinent negatives that you might want to note that appear to contradict your patient's chief complaint. (*Pt complaining of leg numbness, but appears ambulatory without any obvious difficulty. Pt complaining of chest pain, but patient's skin appears warm, pink and dry, while patient appears jovial laughing and talkative with EMS crew asking if he can finish his beer before we take him to hospital.*)

The objective section is without a doubt the shortest of any PCR section as we are limited to what we can see without performing any assessment or diagnostic tests.

A: Assessment- Detail this section the same way that you would write the assessment section of the CHART-E (see chapter 2).

- ABCs or CAB if patient is unresponsive
- Head to toe rapid trauma assessment or same if patient is unconscious or altered
- Focused assessment if injury is isolated
- Lung sounds
- ECG
- 12-Lead
- O2 sat reading
- BGL
- Capnography
- Baseline set of vital signs

Remember to timestamp all your assessment findings and your initial baseline set of vital signs. You may be required, due to patient condition, to initiate rapid transport of a critical patient. If this is the case, continue to finish your physical assessment in this section.

This section should include a Differential Diagnosis (*ddx*) that lends itself to your next section which is your treatment plan. It should also include the statement:

- ***Pt required transport to hospital by ambulance due to...***

If you need to refresh yourself with the importance of including this statement please see Chapter 2. Often times the need for ambulance transport is due to some patient deficit or disability.

Needless to say, being as specific as possible when trying to articulate your patient's condition is tremendously important to your chart.

For example- if your patient presents with contractures, it's not enough just to document, "patient has contractures." You need to be as specific as possible when articulating deficits and disabilities.

- "Pt presented with contractures of the left hand and arm restricting movement, and contractures of the right hand, arm and leg, restricting movement including the ability to ambulate without a wheelchair."
- "Pt presents with left sided hemiparesis affecting patient's arm movement, patient unable to grip anything or maintain elevation of his arm without assistance, and affecting his left leg, making him unambulatory due to being unable to bear weight on his left lower extremity."

P: Treatment Plan- Your plan should be a follow through of what you stated was the differential diagnosis following your assessment. This section will be treatments that you performed on scene as well as those you performed en route to the hospital.

Therefore a timestamp for each intervention becomes extremely important to detail where and when you prioritized your treatments.

And perhaps just as important, who performed the intervention!

- This becomes increasingly important if there are a number of interventions being performed at the same time by different first responders, as is the case with something like a cardiac arrest with ACLS protocols being used.

  -CPR initiated (1902)- Serino
  -BVM @ 15 lpm (1902)- Rogers
  -Defibrillator Pads placed (1904): monitor interpreted as V-Fib- Serino
  -Shock 150j Biphasic (1904)- Summers
  -CPR resumed (1904)- Summers
  -Airway adjunct placed: OPA 90mm (1905)- Rogers
  -Shock 150j Biphasic (1906)- Serino
  -King airway placed: size 4 (1907)- Rogers
  -Advanced airway confirmed and secured (1907)- Serino
  -Shock 150j Biphasic (1908)- Serino
  -IV access 18g Left A/C with Normal Saline running open, 1 attempt/1success (1909)- Summers

Once you have decided to load patient up, you need to clearly mark that down, so there is no ambiguity as to length of time on scene and length of transport.

Be sure to remember what manner you decided to transport patient to the hospital (*code 1 or code 3.*)

And which hospital you decided to transport to. If there is a protocol reason that dictates your decision (*i.e. closest hospital, specialized hospital such as cardiac or stroke center*) be sure to also mark that down.

Time you called the hospital via radio report and dictate any orders you may receive from the hospital. If they give you a room assignment over the radio put that down too.

Once at the hospital be sure to note the time of arrival and the time of patient care turn over.

These are hardly ever the same!

I've arrived at many hospitals only to wait several minutes for a room assignment. When I worked in Las Vegas it was not uncommon, especially on a holiday or a weekend, to sometimes wait close to an hour for a room assignment!

So mark both times down! This is especially true if your times are kept for you by a computer assisted dispatch (CAD) system. The time of arrival to the hospital will be recorded, but the actual time you turn the patient over to the hospital staff will not.

And finally mark down who you turned your patient over to and what their medical title is (*MD, RN*).

E: Exceptions- Again mark down any exceptions that you may have encountered throughout the call that disrupted the flow of your call or were particularly odd.

- Hospital diversions
- Scene became unsafe
- Unable to find patient at dispatched location

SOAP-E example:

S: Medic 5 responding Code 3 for a reported stabbing (2002). Arrived on scene at (2009). Scene secured by APD. Upon our arrival the scene appears to be a private single family residence in a residential neighborhood, noted several broken beer bottles in driveway along with what appears to be blood droplets.

Window on front door appears broken with glass shattered on the outside of the house.

Pt appears to be a male, mid 20's, approximately 70 kg, found lying on his left side on the carpeted floor in the front room.

Pt has what appears to be a white t-shirt wrapped around his left forearm that appears to be saturated with blood. Pt tracking EMS upon approach. Pt states that he was cut by a knife during a fight with his girlfriend, "That bitch stabbed me!"

Pt presents with slurred speech and a strong odor of ETOH coming from his person. Pt admits to consuming "30 beers." There are several empty Budweiser cans thrown around the front room.

Pt states that he has a past medical history of alcohol abuse, consuming approximately 30 beers per day. Pt states that he gets the "shakes" if he stops drinking. Pt denies any further medical history. Pt states that he's supposed to take Prozac for depression but is not compliant with his doctor's orders. Pt cannot remember when he last took this medication. Pt states that he smokes 2 packs of cigarettes a day and smokes marijuana every day. Pt denies any allergies to medications, stating that he is only allergic to "jail."

O: Pt observed to have a patent airway, speaking in multiword sentences without obvious difficulty.

Skin appears warm, pink and dry.

Pt begins to cry stating that he loves his girlfriend but they fight all the time. Pt denies any pain, saying that "I can't feel nothing."

A: Baseline vital signs taken (2012)- Serino P: 110, R: 18, B/P: 110/78, O2 Sat 95%, BGL 102

Pt assessed from head to toe. (2014)- Serino

Pt's face is swollen on the left side, near the eye. Pt admits that his girlfriend threw a can of beer at him and it hit him in the face.

Pt denies any loss of consciousness.

Skull palpated and found to have no signs of trauma.

Neck palpated and visualized: no step offs noted, negative for tracheal deviation or JVD. Clavicles intact.

Chest palpated and visualized: good equal rise and fall with each respiration. Pt able to take in full deep breaths, expanding his intercostal muscles without any difficulty or complaint.

Lung sounds are clear and equal all fields.

Abdominal region palpated in four quadrants with slight tenderness in mid epigastric and RUQ. Pt states "I got a bad liver." Pt states that this tenderness is chronic not acute.

Pelvis palpated and found to be stable.

Posterior visualized and palpated. No trauma noted. Pt has no complaint.

Lower extremities palpated without any complaint or deformity noted. Pt has good PMS in both feet.

Upper extremities, right upper extremity is unremarkable, good radial pulse with appropriate motor and sensory sensation. The left extremity wrapped in t-shirt unwrapped and pt presents with an apparent full thickness laceration on the medial side of the forearm approximately 4" in length. No obvious arterial bleed noted. Pt has good radial pulse and is able to move fingers on left hand without difficulty and has good sensation being able to tell which finger is being touched by EMS. ddx: trauma secondary to stabbing during domestic incident.

Pt requires transport to hospital by ambulance due to blood loss secondary to being stabbed, in addition to patient presenting with signs and symptoms of altered mentation secondary to patient's self-admitted ingestion of multiple alcoholic beverages, along with possible dangerous effects that accompany acute withdrawal.

P: Left arm wrapped in pressure dressing (2016) - Rogers. Distal sensation checked after dressing applied and found to have no compromise. Pt advised to keep arm elevated. Pt lifted to gurney by EMS crew using a commercial patient mover.

Pt positioned in semi fowler on the gurney per patient request for his best position of comfort. Pt transport to UNMH (2020) code 1.

Supplemental oxygen provided, 2 lpm via N/C (2021)- Serino

Pt remained awake and talkative throughout transport. IV access obtained, 18 g right forearm, Normal Saline @ TKO (2025)- Serino

Vital Signs reassessed (2027)- Serino: P: 98, R: 18, B/P 108/76, O2 Sat 98% 2lpm via N/C.

Bandage reassessed with no bleeding through noted.

Hospital Radio Report given (2029)- Serino, Room assignment ER 3. ETA 3 min.

Arrival at Hospital (2032) Patient able to sign PCR chart.

Turned over to Crissy Seifert. RN without incident at (2036). Copy of PCR left with RN.

E: Delay getting to patient until APD secured the scene.

Chapter 4

Narrative Style

For my money the hardest of all EMS charts to write is ironically the one with the least amount of rules.

The narrative format of EMS reports allows its author the freedom to write their chart unencumbered with the restrictions, or expectations that are found when writing using an acronym structured PCR. However, the problems that arise when writing in this style of narrative often come from a lack of style and direction.

I've read many PCR's written in this format that comes across like a body without a skeleton! I'm caught up wading through a massive blob of words and information that lacks any discernable internal structure. This makes the chart appear disorganized and unprofessional.

This is the opposite of what you want!

These charts are often extremely difficult to read through as they can be confusing, misleading and undoubtedly missing key details that probably would have been included had there been more time and organization deployed while writing it out.

Whoa! It does certainly sound like I am not a fan of writing in this format.

And you would be absolutely correct! I am not a fan of the narrative style only PCR.

I think the reason is, like most EMS providers I've met, I tend to be more of a Type A personality: someone who likes to stay in control of things, in this case the narrative. When I'm reading someone else's report, I want to have some idea their chart is going to answer the questions I need answered.

It's just a matter of preference.

Now with that disclaimer out of the way, there certainly is a way to write a strong EMS chart using the narrative style format; it just requires practice and learning three rules!

Rule #1- The Narrative format does not equate to freeform!

I've read and critiqued a large number of EMS charts that appear to be just scattered bits of information with no connective flow.

Pt is a male c/o of stomach hurting for three days, daughter states that she ate birthday cake a week ago and thinks it might have gone bad. The house is unkempt and has alcohol bottles everywhere. Pt states he vomited three times yesterday and two times today. He states he thinks he may be dying. Pt can't remember if he ate one or two pieces of birthday cake but did not think it went bad. The wife ate some and the daughter too. The patient states that he's had no bowel movements for three days.

He's not sure if his vomit had blood in it. Pt states he drinks alcohol every day, but did not have money to buy any today. Pt is diaphoretic with rapid pulse. He is allergic to aspirin and penicillin. He rates his pain a 10 out of 10 in severity but cannot remember when it got to this elevated level of pain. He states his foot also....etc....

Um... huh?

I wouldn't know if this patient was suffering from food poisoning, ETOH withdrawals, or something else totally unrelated.

Your PCR is not a notepad for you to jot down random thoughts and tidbits of information as you happen to remember them. It is still a legal document that needs to be carefully arranged in order to address all audiences who will be looking at it.

Rule #2- Use Chronology as a way to keep your PCR organized!

Timestamp important events throughout your call and let them serve as markers for your PCR. For example, use the time you were dispatched and the time you arrived as timestamp markers. Then you simply can fill in the gaps in the middle. The more timestamps you utilize, the more organized your chart will appear to be.

- *Medic 4 dispatched (1918) for 18 y/o male ejection from vehicle, possibly other victims on scene. Medic 4 responded code 3, requested additional resources in the area, requested air transport to meet us on scene. Arrived on scene (1923) Medic 4 first on scene establishing incident command.*

- *Baseline Vital signs taken- Serino (0814). Rapid head to toe physical assessment performed- Rogers, patient found to have several abrasions and road rash on left arm, left hand and left axial chest and abdomen (0816). Pt logrolled onto right side by EMS crew and Fire Dept Crew, Pt found to have extensive abrasions on posterior including thoracic, lumbar and buttocks. Clean sterile dressing placed on abrasions prior to pt being placed on backboard (0817)- Serino. Pt placed on backboard (0818) PMS assessed x 4 extremities prior to securing to backboard found to have no deficits- Rogers, Pt secured to backboard immobilizing C-spine (0820), PMS checked x 4 extremities without deficits.- Rogers.*

For those of you who think this might be overkill, remember that often we are on scene for only 10 minutes or so. In this time we might generate 8-12 timestamps? Not really a lot if we are trying to accurately document what we did on scene. And of course not everything we do is going to generate a timestamp, but we should always be open to the idea that the more we do produce, the more details we are able to give, the more the reader of your PCR is going to be able to understand what you faced and the challenges you had to overcome.

Rule #3- Break up your PCR into logical paragraphs!

Nothing is as daunting as being asked to read a PCR that looks like one long, unending paragraph. We want our PCRs to be easy to read and easy to understand. Trying to discern specific details and interventions out of wall of words is difficult. Our eyes will oftentimes start to gloss over and someone might just skim over an important detail that might be useful to help our patient, our company or yourself. Try giving yourself your own natural breakers, using chronology to group together certain parts of your chart so they're easy to follow and understand.

For instance:

- DISPATCH
- ON SCENE
- TRANSPORT
- TURN OVER.

Depending on how much information you obtain, you might want to break up the PCR even further. This will especially be apt for the On Scene and Transport portions of your chart which logically will be where you put the bulk of your information.

Narrative style: example:

Medic 6 dispatched to 3679 Stornoway Dr, for a 69 year old female altered mentation. Per dispatch information, patient's husband activated 911 when he noticed his wife not acting like herself (0649).

Upon our arrival (0652), met by patient's husband at door. Residential neighborhood, house appears well maintained and shows no signs of disarray. Husband led EMS to master bedroom where patient is sitting on edge of bed.

At patient at side (0653) patient appears approximately 85 kg, awake and tracks EMS but does not respond to EMS introductions. No immediate life threats noted.

Vital signs taken by Serino (0655): Pt airway: patent. Breathing: 14 bpm unlabored, with equal chest rise and fall with each respiration. Circulation: Skin WPD, pulse 78, irregular and strong at radial.

According to husband, patient and he went to bed last night at 2200 with no complaints from patient. "Everything was normal," according to pt's husband. Husband woke up at 0600 and patient did not appear to respond to their alarm, which she normally does. He tried to wake her at 0630. He did not have trouble waking her, but she presented with aphasia.

FAST-G performed- Rogers (0656) No signs of facial droop. No arm drift. Pt is aphasic. Weak grip left side. Glucose 129.

Rule out: CVA. Notification of stroke alert- Serino (0659). Pt lifted by EMS crew to gurney. Pt does not appear to be able to nod or shake her head to communicate pain or discomfort.

Pt's husband agreed to come with EMS to hospital via ambulance. Pt's husband states patient has not recently incurred any trauma, no recent changes in medications, or any recent radical changes in diet or exercise. Husband does state that they both just came back yesterday from a long drive, approximately 12 hours, driving back from their son's graduation in New Orleans. Husband is uncertain if patient is compliant with her medications.

Pt, according to husband, has a medical history of A-fib, hypertension and migraine headaches. She takes metoprolol, warfarin, and Lanoxin. He is not certain what patient takes for migraine.

Pt has NKDA.

Transport initiated (0705) code 3 to Presbyterian hospital.

Physical exam: eyes PERRL, Neck: midline, no sign of tracheal deviation or JVD. Chest: lung sounds clear and equal all fields. Abdomen: soft, no signs of tenderness from patient's face upon palpation. Extremities x 4: no signs of edema, strong pulses.

Vital Signs- Serino (0710) Pulse 76 @ R radial, B/P 180/92, Resp: 18.

Radio Report sent advising patient's current condition. No orders received from receiving hospital – Serino (0712).

Vital Signs- Serino (0715) Pulse 79 @ R radial, B/P 178.94, Resp: 18.

Arrived at Hospital (0718).

Pt taken directly to Room 1 and met by ER staff. Pt sheeted off gurney and onto hospital bed by ER and EMS staff.

Pt report given to RN Karen Otzenberger- Serino (0721). Copy of PCR left with RN.

Chapter 5

Ambiguity and Contradictions

Hopefully, after reading the last three chapters you can appreciate just how much raw information and specific details you can cram into each patient care report. Always keep in mind that every PCR you write should help to present an accurate picture that allows the reader to see just how you evaluated, assessed and treated your patient.

And the way you do that is with details and information. Try to think of each detail or piece of information as a single paint stroke on a much larger canvas The more paint strokes you choose to apply, the more vivid and realistic the picture you are trying to create will appear to be.

Remember, we are shooting for clarity not ambiguity, so an accurate presentation of what you did should be your best defense if anyone ever questions what you did, or decided not to do.

However, for every piece of information you decide to include, you increase the risk of ambiguity and contradiction somewhere down the road.

Of course this is bad. And somewhat ironic!

A detail or piece of information you hoped might clarify your treatment or solidify your thought process can suddenly become a stumbling block that might derail the credibility of your entire chart. This is especially true if a chart with inconsistencies is ever presented one day in a court of law. Lawyers and paralegals get paid lots of money to scrutinize medical charts looking for this very thing.

Just remember that the more information you include and the more details you decide to document, the higher the risk you run of contradicting yourself somewhere else in your chart!

However this should never stop you from documenting as much information as you can. It should give you pause to double check what you have written to ensure there is nothing that doesn't add up.

And while of course contradicting yourself or writing something that isn't consistent is never your intention it does occasionally happen. In fact there are a number of ways an EMS provider can accomplish this during the course of writing a detailed chart.

In fact, you might find that maintaining consistency and avoiding contradictions throughout the course of writing your chart may be one of the most difficult skills to master.

Try to follow these five rules to help you avoid documenting unintended mistakes.

1. **Look for areas of possible redundancy!**
   Depending on the charting program your
   company or department is using, chances are
   there are a number of areas that are required to
   be filled in for statistical purposes or for
   research data. This often equates to filling in
   your vital signs, level of consciousness and
   specific diagnostic procedures: i.e. BGL, SpO2,
   Capnography, or medication interventions to be
   included in a drop down section, as well as
   included in your narrative. This is one of the
   most common areas for inconsistencies to take
   place. For example, in one area you might have
   documented that the patient has a GCS of 15, but
   in another place you document that he is
   confused or showing signs of being responsive
   only to painful stimuli. Or you might document
   that the patient's blood pressure is one reading,
   but in your narrative it might be something else.
   Redundancy should never be something that you
   fear or try to avoid; rather it is simply a matter of
   accurately documenting the correct information.
   Timestamping your interventions and vital signs
   is one way I've found to help ensure that not only
   you will avoid contradicting yourself, but also
   more accurately document the correct time you
   performed these interventions.

2. **Don't procrastinate! Write your chart as soon as your call is over.** This may be easier said than done, especially if you happen to be working in a busy system. Until you are comfortable with writing your charts with numerous distractions, I would recommend you find a quiet spot by yourself to help you write out your chart. Use the notes that you have taken throughout the course of your chart and get started.

    Procrastination is your mortal enemy when it comes to writing clear, articulate charts that do not have errors in consistency.

    The sooner you write your chart, the more accurate your recollection of the events will be. You may remember a detail that is vitally important and may have been lost if you waited to write it out. The more you write, the more comfortable you will become with putting your thoughts down on paper. And with greater frequency will hopefully come greater speed. However, this brings up a great point that most modern ambulance and fire departments require their medical charts to be typed out, either into a portable Toughbook style computer, or on a PCR back at the station. This means that the faster you are able to type, the faster you will be able to dictate the thoughts in your head onto the blank computer screen in front of you. So if typing is a weak spot for you, either you do not know how to type and are forced to pick at the keyboard, or do not type very fast, you may find it a worthwhile investment to take a typing course at a local community college, or buy yourself a typing program that you can use to help increase your speed. Believe me, being able to type with a greater speed is a benefit that will more than pay for itself in the long run.

3. **Learn to proofread your material!**
Proofreading is a skill that must be practiced in order for it to be effective. It is often difficult to scrutinize something you just have written, but I highly recommend that you do. Look especially for areas that you know are potential thorns that might snag threads of consistency. Vital signs and level of consciousness are two of the biggest areas where people might be susceptible to inconsistencies. Ask yourself what your patient's mentation is throughout the course of the call and does the documented GCS or LOC remain consistent with what you are reporting? Just as you are required in reassessment to start from the very beginning and recheck LOC and ABC's you should be doing this with your documented vital signs and mentation. It's easy to put vital signs into one area of drop down boxes and without even thinking you are documenting the patient's mentation is showing no signs of being altered. But the patient's presentation in the

chart says something quite different. If you have a patient that does indeed have altered mentation, be very careful to correlate areas of redundancy to ensure they match up. Again, as stated in previous chapters, this is one area that lawyers are especially apt at finding. With each instance of inconsistency, you further erode your credibility as a capable and competent first responder.

4. **Consistency in reporting.** As boring as this might sound, I've found that if I write my charts the exact same way each time, I limit the areas that might get me into trouble. By developing my own pattern of style, I'm able to speed up the time it takes for me to write my chart, while limiting the areas of inconsistency and contradictions. This style does not eliminate the need for me to proofread my document, nor does it guarantee that I might contradict myself in certain areas. However, what it does mean is that hopefully I will be more successful at catching these unintended errors before I submit my chart and can no longer alter it without adding an addendum. I've mentioned that I've had to learn to alter my style somewhat depending on which service I'm working for. For example, in New Mexico, where I spent the bulk of my EMS career, the prevalent narrative format style was C.H.A.R.T. It was a style I got used to and became

very fast at writing. When I moved to Florida, I found that most services here used the S.O.A.P. format so I needed to slightly alter my way of documenting. However, once I did, I was back to writing my charts the exact same way in order to ensure that I felt comfortable writing my charts quickly, while at the same time not missing any pieces of information I knew I wanted to include into my report.

5. **Don't use terms that assume a patient's condition.** Several acronyms and phrases have become almost commonplace in medical terminology are predicated on the assumption of the EMS crew knowing what the patient is feeling. Terms such as:

...placed patient in best position of comfort

...patient is bedridden

...PUTS (patient unable to sign)

And perhaps my least favorite phrase *...within normal limits*

Each of these phrases is commonly written without any substantial evidence that indicates we understand what it means.

How do we know what is the position of best comfort for a patient we have just met?

Patient is bedridden? Can she not ambulate? Is this a medical or physical condition? Does she have both legs or is there an amputation that you did not chart?

Patient is unable to sign? Why? Did they not have a pen? Did they have a medical or physical condition you were not treating? Did the patient refuse to sign?

And when it comes to the phrase *within normal limits* you are comparing your patient to a **relative normal** found only in textbooks. If you happen to find a patient with a heart rate of 52, this might be outside of the normal relative range that most textbooks refer to. But taken in context, the patient is a long distance bicyclist and marathon runner and his normal resting heart rate is 50, well then this heart rate is *within the **patient's** normal limits!*

Look for common phrases that assume rather than illustrate what we are trying to write about the patient we are treating and documenting. These are common sources of ambiguity that can be made by a savvy attorney to make it seem like you did a poor patient assessment.

If you find yourself wanting to write a phrase such as this, stop and ask yourself, *Is there a better way I can write this that explains what I'm writing rather than assumes?*

Chapter 6

Patient Assessment & Pertinent Negatives

As I stated in the introduction of this book, we as first responders have a responsibility to perform four basic tasks when it comes to each and every call we respond to:

1. To assess our patient by learning their chief complaint, acquiring their medical history and performing a physical examination.

2. We need to intelligently make a differential diagnosis based on the results of our patient assessment.

3. We need to treat our patient with interventions and transport based on the results of our differential diagnosis.

4. And we need to document all aspects of our call in order to benefit:
   a. The patient
   b. The profession
   c. The provider

Everything starts with the patient assessment!

From the moment I'm dispatched and told what I am responding to, I'm starting to make a mental list in my head of possible causes, or as I like to think of them, suspects, that might be the guilty culprit for the problem at hand. I'm thinking about what I might find and what I might need to accomplish in the short amount of time I am with my patient.

For anyone who's played chess, it's similar to trying to think two or three moves ahead, so I can plan my strategy of attack.

For example, if I'm dispatched to a chest pain call, I'm thinking:

- Acute Coronary Syndrome (MI). I usually try to start with what is the worst case scenario and list that first.
- Cardiac Tamponade
- Chest Trauma
- Endocarditis
- Angina
- Pulmonary Embolism

So there is a rapid list of six possible suspects that could easily be the cause of my patient's chest pain.

Of course there could be a reason you haven't listed!

But at least you have an idea of what it might be and what you would do in each of these situations.

Once on scene, I try to be hyper tune my awareness of my surroundings, both as a safety issue and in order to start gathering information. So in essence, my patient assessment starts the moment I arrive on scene.

Everything from the condition of the patient's house, how they were found, their level of consciousness, their chief complaint, medical history and physical examination needs to be carefully looked at and evaluated in order to come up with a presumptive differential diagnosis.

If the patient is awake and talking to you, you can start by introducing yourself to the patient. If they respond appropriately, then you have a better idea of your patient's level of consciousness as well as their **airway** patency. You can then assess your patient's **breathing**, *rate depth and quality*, as well as their **circulation**, *pulse rate, regularity, strength, skin color, temperature and condition.*

All the while you should be making notes to aid in our ability to most accurately document our findings and interventions. I would caution against jotting down notes on your gloves, which although they are convenient to write on, are quickly discarded and vital information easily lost. Use a reporter's notebook, a large piece of 2" tape placed on your thigh to write down your observations.

However you do it, begin by training yourself to take notes throughout the call!

A patient history and physical examination both yield a tremendous amount of information about the patient and your decisions on a course of action. Do not rely on your memory to retain this much information that you are receiving at such a rapid rate. It's almost impossible to remember that much detail without taking notes.

The ability to write down information as you get it is a valuable skill that will require practice. However, you can take comfort in knowing that only you need to understand your notes! Nobody else is going to be reading them; so write them in a way that is best for YOU to understand. Don't be ashamed if your notes are messy, or nobody else can read or understand them. Nobody else has to; these notes are for you to be able to transcribe into a professional document at the end of the call.

If you patient is unconscious or has an altered level of consciousness, you are going to have to perform a thorough head to toe assessment to look for any DCAP-BTLS:

- *D: Deformities/Distention*
- *C: Contusions/Crepitus*
- *A: Abrasions*
- *P: Punctures*

- ***B: Burns***
- ***T: Tenderness***
- ***L: Lacerations***
- ***S: Swelling***

Remember, if your patient cannot tell you something with words, they may be able to tell you something with presentation.

Medical necklaces, bracelets, track marks on the arms, pinpoint pupils, vomit, empty pill bottles, bruising, hives, or something found in a patient's medicine cabinet, might be just the clue you need to help you more effectively treat your patient.

Use your diagnostic skills such as taking a BGL, performing a 12-lead ECG, and placing the patient on capnography to better help you narrow down the list of possible suspects you formulated in your head, until you've settled on just one or two. This will be your differential diagnosis and this should be how you proceed to treat your patient.

One additional tool you can deploy to help you narrow down your list of possible suspects is your ability to recognize a **pertinent negative**!

A pertinent negative is something that you might expect to find during your patient history or assessment, based on the patient's chief complaint, but for some reason or another is not present or the patient denies.

60-year old female complaining of severe shortness of breath meets EMS at the front door holding a cigarette and speaking in multi-word sentences without obvious signs of dyspnea. Pt states she is having difficulty breathing, however she is ambulating unassisted, skin is warm, pink and dry and she is laughing at the questions posed to her by EMS crew. Pt denies any recent cough, fatigue or exertional dyspnea. Pt begins to cry and states she has been extremely lonely since her husband passed away last month. Lung sounds clear and equal all fields. SpO2 reading is 97% on room air.

In order for it to be considered a **pertinent negative** it must in some way be associated with the patient's chief complaint.

So in the above scenario, we have a female who is complaining of severe shortness of breath however is not displaying typical signs or symptoms that might be associated with someone who has her chief complaint.

Typically, someone who is complaining of severe dyspnea cannot speak in multi-word sentences, does not have clear lung sounds, warm, pink and dry skin, an SpO2 reading above 96% and would most likely be fatigued or complaining of exertional dyspnea. Therefore all of these would be considered relevant and pertinent negatives based on the patient's chief complaint.

The fact that patient had a cigarette in her hand, or is recently widowed is not necessarily a pertinent negative, but they are relevant findings that should also be included in the documentation.

If the patient throughout the assessment denies back pain or diabetes, these are not necessarily pertinent negatives because back pain and diabetes are not typically associated with a complaint of shortness of breath.

Therefore, our differential diagnosis might change from something like respiratory distress to something more akin to emotional distress and our treatment and transport decisions might change because of this.

Remember though, unless you choose to document all of your findings, including the pertinent negatives, a good portion of your patient assessment will be lost and your treatment decisions may also be called into question.

Pertinent negatives are also an effective tool to solidify your diagnosis enabling you to justify deploying certain interventions or the reasons behind withholding certain interventions or procedures.

Another example of a scenario that has pertinent negatives would be:

48 y/o male complaining of severe abdominal pain for over one week. Pt found lying on the ground guarding his abdomen with both knees flexed towards his chest. Pt denies any nausea or vomiting, denies any recent changes in diet or medications. Pt admits to several problems with bowel movements, including black tarry stools and the appearance of blood in his stool. Upon examination patient has pain in the upper quadrants with patient stating it is greater in the upper right quadrant. Pt's skin and sclera appear slightly jaundiced. Pt denies any alcohol consumption and denies a past history of alcohol abuse or hepatitis. Pt states that he still has his appendix and gallbladder. An empty ½ gallon bottle of vodka was found in the patient's kitchen in his trash can; however patient denies being the one who consumed it. Pt does not present with slurred speech but does have a noticeable odor of possible ETOH on his breath. Pt states he was assaulted last week in an attempted robbery and was punched in the abdomen repeatedly by the assailants. No signs of bruising or discoloration noted upon visual examination of the patient's abdomen.

Whew! There is a slew of relevant information found in that paragraph, including some pertinent negatives mixed in with other important pieces of information.

Let's break it down piece by piece!

- The way the patient was found, lying on the floor with knees flexed towards the chest, is to be expected from someone who is complaining of severe abdominal pain. If this patient had been found walking around without obvious pain, this would have been a pertinent negative, but seeing as how he matches what we would expect- let's move on.

- Pt denies any nausea or vomiting: this is our first pertinent negative as these would be two symptoms that we normally would associate with severe abdominal pain.
- Pt denies any recent changes in diet or medications: two more important pieces of information that may be the possible cause of abdominal pain. So these are most certainly pertinent negatives.
- Pt admits to several problems with his bowel movements. Again, these are to be expected in someone with abdominal pain as the cause could very well have something to do with a problem with the gastrointestinal tract. If he had denied any such problems, these would be pertinent negatives.
- Pain in the upper right quadrant of the abdomen is not a pertinent negative as this is very much something we might expect in someone with this chief complaint.
- Skin and sclera are jaundiced. This doesn't necessarily sound like something that might fit into a patient's chief complaint of abdominal pain, but with the surrounding clues we will acquire, it most certainly is a relevant piece to possibly solving this puzzle.
- Pt states he still has his appendix and gallbladder. Two organs that can easily become

enflamed and cause abdominal pain. If the patient had these organs removed at some point in the past, we could rule them out as possible suspects. Since he hasn't, they remain possible culprits.

- A large empty bottle of vodka found in the patient's trash can in the kitchen. Chronic alcohol abuse could most certainly fit the signs of jaundice and the symptoms of abdominal pain in the upper right quadrant where the liver is located. However, the patient denies consuming the alcohol. Which makes this is a most interesting pertinent negative, because alcohol abuse seems to coming into focus as the most likely suspect to cause this patient's problems. This patient may be embarrassed by his predicament and chose to fib about a possible personal problem. Either way, the bottle is included into the report.

- Pt does not have slurred speech, but does have an odor of possible ETOH on his breath. The negative slurred speech is now a pertinent negative as the focus on alcohol abuse is being focused on. The odor of possible ETOH is a carefully worded sentence that is meant to convey that while I smell something that I recognize as probably alcohol on this patient's breath: I'm not an expert on this subject, so I included the word *possible ETOH*, to indicate this. Never paint yourself into a corner by using specific words in your documentation- unless you are 100% certain you can back it up with either diagnostic tests or the patient admits to something.

- And last, the patient states that he was assaulted last week and struck in the abdomen. This could most certainly explain the patient's condition. However, the notation that there was no sign of bruising or discoloration seen upon visual examination therefore becomes another pertinent negative.

Being able to perform a thorough patient assessment is one of the most vital parts of any EMS call. It is where a tremendous amount of questions is asked and a virtual avalanche of information is learned. However, just as important is your ability to document your findings and interventions.

Don't allow yourself to be buried under the amount of details and information you are about to receive. Keep yourself afloat by maintaining notes throughout the call. Try to train yourself to look for the unusual elements you might find throughout the call. Sometimes something as seemingly benign as a patient's clothing, or what may or may not be in a patient's refrigerator might be relevant to the narrative you are trying to tell. It's oftentimes the little details that make the biggest impact to the reader. It just all depends on how you, the provider, perceive the situation and wish to document your findings.

It's important to get the pertinent patient information as soon as you can: name (with correct spelling), age, chief complaint, past medical history, etc. Then you can focus on assessment and interventions and transport. Pertinent negatives are effective at helping you narrow down your list of potential suspects until you have one or two best guesses for your differential diagnosis.

Remember, you are not just documenting what the patient complained about and how they presented upon your arrival, you are also justifying your decisions and clarifying why you performed some procedures, while holding off on others. Your documentation serves to benefit not just the patient, but you the provider as you will both be looked at evaluated in one way or another.

Chapter 7

Patient Refusals

I've never been one to look at patient refusals as an easy call. Sure we may escape the time spent transporting a patient. However it didn't take long for me to learn that whatever time I gained by not transporting my patient was instead spent logging vital signs, details and information into my patient refusal. I soon began to **hate** taking patient refusals, simply because I knew the amount of time I would soon be spending writing out this incredibly detailed and complex report.

And now, with over 20 years of EMS experience behind me, I can most assuredly state that out of all the different types of EMS narratives I was required to write; I found none more challenging than documenting the patient refusal.

And the reason for this is simple... **LIABILITY!**

As first responders we have a **DUTY TO ACT:** which means we have a legal obligation to respond to a patient who requests our help, regardless of race, gender, sexual orientation, or their ability to pay for services. Once we respond, we have to do our due diligence in performing an assessment and offering transport to a hospital, no matter what the situation.

As first responders we should never dissuade a patient from going to the hospital if they want to! EVER!!!

That's not our job.

Our job is to treat the patients we respond to as professionals, offering them a safe and expeditious transport to the hospital; not to make judgement calls on the validity of whether someone does or does not need an ambulance.

So when faced with a patient who wants to refuse transport to the hospital, it raises a number of legal questions that need to be thoroughly addressed before this can happen.

So first and foremost, a patient who is competent and understands the risks involved with refusing transport **ABSOLUTELY** has the right to sign a refusal.

So then the number one priority becomes how you document this.

If you respond to a patient who wishes to refuse EMS transport, you are then tasked with:

- Performed a detailed medical assessment
- Determined that your patient is competent to make his own decisions
- And thoroughly had the risks of refusing transport explained to them

99

- Documenting your findings in a way that display that you have met all three of these criteria.

Determining competency can be difficult, but documenting it in a way that a reader can understand might be even harder!

DON'T BE VAGUE; BE AS SPECIFIC AS YOU CAN!

Writing out specific details takes time and effort. However when dealing with a patient refusal you are always building a case to defend yourself in the event anything happens to this patient after you leave. Because if an attorney finds out that his client was hurt or died soon after being medically evaluated by a first responder and allowed to sign a refusal, your chart is being subpoenaed faster than you can say Atticus Finch.

So the name of the game is specifics.

A quick way to gage a patient's competency is by assessing to see if they are alert and oriented to themselves, their surroundings and their current condition. Most first responders discover this by asking a certain number of questions that, if answered correctly by the patient, would lend credence to their decision making ability.

Typically abbreviated AxO, alert and oriented is followed by the number of questions asked to gage how oriented the patient is: AxO x 3 or AxO x 4, etc.

Usually you want to ask questions that gage both a patient's short term awareness and long term awareness.

It's not enough to write something generic such as: **Pt was AxO x 3,** as a catchall for documenting competency.

> **ATTORNEY**: *"AxO x 3? What does that mean?"*

> **PARAMEDIC**: *"Um... my patient was alert and oriented times 3."*

> **ATTORNEY**: *"3? Three what?"*

> **PARAMEDIC**: *"Person, Place and Time."*

> **ATTORNEY**: *"And how did you determine this.? Did the patient know the city he was in? The state? How about the planet? And the time, did your patient know the exact time when you asked? The day? The year? How about the century? Mr. Paramedic, we may never know the exact answer to this because it isn't documented in your report is that true?"*

> **PARAMEDIC**: *"I usually ask my patient the city..."*

> **ATTORNEY**: *"I usually sleep on the left side of the bed. Sometimes the right. Sometimes I can't remember what side I slept on. So things change, situations change, and memories fade, is that not correct sir?"*

Hopefully you get the picture. The more vague you are in your documentation, the more you leave the door open for a lawyer to interpret the narrative for you.

Take the time to write out what your patient is oriented to and what they are not oriented to.

ex. *Patient was oriented to his name, today's date and why EMS was called.*

This brief documentation leaves little doubt to what the patient was asked and what the patient's responses were.

DOCUMENT THE RISKS RELAYED TO PATIENT!

In order for a patient to make an informed refusal, he has to be informed of the risks he faces by refusing transport by EMS, as well as the benefits he would gain if he accepted transport.

This is another area of ambiguity that attorneys love to sniff around. Why you may ask? Because often times a first responder will write something generic such as:

Patient was informed of the risks of refusing EMS transport.

This is never enough information. By now after hopefully reading the previous chapters, you can imagine how an attorney would find a way to corrupt the intent of this EMS chart.

ATTORNEY: *"Your patient was complaining of severe chest pain. And yet you allowed him to sign a refusal after you evaluated him."*

PARAMEDIC: *"Yes."*

ATTORNEY: *"The chart states you informed the patient of the risks and benefits of refusing EMS transport."*

PARAMEDIC: *"Yes sir, it does."*

ATTORNEY: *"Does that mean you informed the patient of all possible, conceivable risks he may face by refusing transport."*

PARAMEDIC: *"Well maybe not all."*

ATTORNEY: *"Some? Would that be fair to say?"*

PARAMEDIC: *"Yes."*

ATTORNEY: *"Perhaps what you happened to remember that day. Or the ones you thought were most important. We'll leave some in, but not others. Well there is no way to really tell can we by reading this chart as it doesn't actually state what you informed your patient about. Let me ask you, did you inform my client, your patient, of the possibility of a cardiac tamponade?"*

PARAMEDIC: *"I advised him that there might be something cardiac in nature."*

ATTORNEY: *"Where is that written in the chart? My client does not remember you mentioning anything about his problem being cardiac in nature."*

PARAMEDIC: *"Of course I did."*

Hands the paramedic the chart.

ATTORNEY: *"Please show me where in your chart you state that. "*

GAME OVER

Now of course this might be an over simplified version of what might happen in a courtroom, but I hope it makes a point of how details and lack of details can make a difference.

I'm sure any first responder who is faced with an obvious problem, such as an acute coronary syndrome would absolutely inform their patient of the possibility of a myocardial infarction, along with other cardiac and respiratory problems. But if they are not specifically written out in your chart, well... as an old English proverb once said, ***"Hell is paved with good intentions."***

Specify the risks you are concerned with.

If it is a cardiac problem, document clearly in your chart that you warned your patient he could be having a cardiac event which could result in serious injury or even possibly death.

Remember, we do our best as first responders to offer an assessment and a possible differential diagnosis, so use this as your guide to what you should be warning your patient about.

This is especially true if your patient is signing a refusal, against medical advice. If you have a patient that is, despite your best efforts and verbal judo, will not go with you to the hospital. Remember to clearly document exactly what it is you are worried about, i.e. *MI, CVA, Intracranial Bleed, etc.* Document that you explained the specific risks the patient is facing if he does not come into the hospital with you, i.e. *paralysis, respiratory failure, death, etc.*

And if at all possible, explain this to your patient in the presence of a witness. This way you can have them sign off on your chart that, you did indeed explain the areas of your concern to your patient.

Having a witness, preferably one who is a family member to the patient can be a crucial piece of evidence when it comes to defending your chart in a courtroom.

If you can't get someone related to the patient, then use a friend of the patient, a police officer, a firefighter, and last resort, your partner. And, I say last resort, simply because if anyone would be perceived by a jury as having a possible reason to lie for you, it would be someone you work with. But still, anyone is better than no one.

PUTTING IT ALL TOGETHER

Upon your arrival you should immediately determine your patient's chief complaint, either from the patient's own words or through the circumstances you find them in.

Perform your primary and secondary assessment. Take the time to get a thorough medical history, including your SAMPLE, OPQRST.

Get at least two sets of vital signs. One set of vital signs is merely a snapshot of your patient's condition at one point in time. It tells you very little. However, compared to another set of vital signs and now you are getting a trend of the patient's condition. Is he getting better or worse, stable or unstable, sick or not sick?

Make a specific differential diagnosis if you can, based on your patient assessment and medical history. This will allow you to think about your course of action if you *were* to take your patient to the hospital. Offering to tell your patient the benefits of going in by ambulance might just be enough to sway them to accepting transport.

A differential diagnosis will also allow you to speak in specifics when you are addressing the risks involved when your patient refuses transport.

EMS REFUSAL EXAMPLE

S: Medic 51 responded Code 3 for an apparent diabetic emergency. Arrived on scene at (2018). Upon our arrival scene appears to be a large multi-family apartment complex. Pt lives on third floor. No elevator so stair chair brought up with EMS equipment. Met at front door by patient's wife who led EMS to back bedroom where patient found (2020) laying supine in bed, not responsive to initial EMS approach.

Pt is a 37 y/o male, approximately 80 kg, responsive only to painful stimuli. According to patient's wife she had returned home from work and found her husband lying unresponsive in bed. According to patient's wife he is a poor manager of his diabetes who apparently "does this all the time."

In addition to patient's Type I diabetes, patient has a past medical history of hypertension. Pt has NKDA. Pt takes Insulin and Metoprolol, both of which according to patient's wife he is non-compliant with.

O: Pt has a patent airway and is breathing non labored. Skin appears pale with signs of slight diaphoresis. Room appears to be clean and well maintained. Pt appears to be groomed with no obvious signs of lack of personal hygiene or signs of abuse noted.

A: Initial vitals taken by Rogers at (2023) P: 116, B/P: 138/88, Resp: 18, Lung Sounds Clear/Equal, Skin: pale and clammy, O2 sat 96%, BGL: 23.

IV established by Serino at (2028) 18g in patient's left A/C 1 attempt/1success, NS with a 500 cc fluid challenge.

25g of Dextrose 50% SIVP- Serino (2031).

Head to toe physical exam performed, no signs of trauma noted save for pt's left hand which is heavily bandaged from what patient's wife describes as a previous incident at patient's work: paralegal, patient caught his hand in a pinch point.

At (2037) Pt opened his eyes and began to look around at EMS. Pt was initially confused as to the situation he found himself in, but he appeared to quickly grasp why EMS was there without us having to tell him. "I did it again, didn't I?"

Vital signs taken (2040)- Rogers. P 108 Strong and Regular, B/P 142/86, Resp: 18 , Lung Sounds

Clear/Equal, Skin pale and clammy, O2 sat 97%, BGL 139.

Pt given a few minutes to further orientate himself. Wife explained to him that he again forgot to eat after taking his insulin.

Pt's wife handed him a peanut butter and jelly sandwich with some orange juice to drink.

At (2045) Pt states that he is in no pain. Pt is oriented to his name; he knows the current date and what city he is in. He is able to relate what happened: he got busy on the phone with work and forgot to eat the dinner his wife left for him. Pt's wife works nights.

Pt states that he does not want to go to the hospital by ambulance.

Pt advised, with his wife present, that poorly managed diabetes is a tremendous health risk. The possibility that he could go into a diabetic coma could result in permanent damage or even death.

It is strongly advised to patient and to his wife that they accept the ambulance ride to the hospital where he can be further evaluated to ensure no damage has been done and his lab work can be drawn and confirmed.

Pt advises that he has a doctor's appointment tomorrow with his own personal physician and that he would prefer to wait until then.

Pt's wife states that she is off until tomorrow afternoon and she will be here with the patient in order to ensure that he eats and takes his medications as he is supposed to.

Vital signs taken at (2055)- Rogers. P: 98, B/P: 134/82, Resp: 16, Skin: WPD, O2 Sat: 98%, BGL: 131.

Patient again offered and advised to accept medical transport from EMS. Patient states that he appreciates the offer but is going to refuse. Pt asked to read the patient refusal form and sign it.

Pt's wife was on hand throughout and asked to sign as a witness that patient is refusing transport against medical advice. Pt states that she understands the severity of the problem and the possible risks and benefits that were relayed to her by EMS.

She signed the refusal (2103)

IV was D/C'ed – Serino (2105) Pt and his wife informed that they can call us back at any time if they feel the need to. Both state they understand and thanked us for our service.

EMS cleared scene and back in service (2111)

Chapter 8

Transporting a Patient Against Their Will

One of the most critical decisions an EMT or paramedic will have to make at some point throughout their career is: *Am I going to have to transport my patient to the hospital against their will?*

Taking away a patient's right to refuse transport and transporting them against their will is a serious, sometimes hostile, event that will have to be documented thoroughly.

However, before we can even start to think about documenting, we have to be able to determine *why* we are choosing to take this aggressive measure.

Basically, there are really only three reasons why you would want to take a patient's right to refuse treatment and transport away from them:

1. Your patient, after you have assessed them, does not appear to be oriented to the point where they can fully understand the risks of being allowed to refuse transport.

2. They have made statements that indicate some sort of suicidal ideation or have actually attempted to harm themselves in a suicide attempt.

3. The patient is a minor.

In each of these situations there is ample opportunity for two variations of the truth to be found. The patient who you have chosen to take to the hospital against their wishes might remember the scene a whole lot different from the way you do.

So again the devil is in the details when it comes to how you are going to document this chart. The less details, the more open you are for your narrative to be interpreted in a way you neither intended nor wanted. The key thing to remember is to document **specific** reasons why you decided to transport your patient against their wishes.

Of the three reasons listed above the first is usually the one most open to interpretation. You may have to use your words to illustrate what exactly you found that lead you to believe your patient was incapable of making an informed refusal.

Did your patient appear intoxicated? If so why?

Did your patient display slurred speech when answering your questions?

Was there an odor of ETOH coming off the person?

Did they present with a staggered gait?

Was there evidence of possible drug use? If so, what was it?

Was the patient not able to answer your questions appropriately?

Was there a delay in his responses that seemed odd or out of place?

Does your patient have a history of being intellectually delayed?

Does your patient have a psych history?

Are they non-compliant with their medications?

Is your patient oriented to himself and his surroundings? If not, what is he confused about?

Does your patient have a history of dementia or displaying signs of delirium?

Is your patient acting appropriate for the situation at hand?

It is up to **you** the EMS provider who is documenting this PCR to make the case that in your opinion this patient needed to go the hospital and they could not reasonably sign a refusal. In order to make this case you have to be able to anticipate what questions your reader might have and provide enough details and information to convincingly answer them.

More specifically, think about what an attorney hired by an upset patient, who you transported against their will, might be looking for.

The other two reasons are pretty straight forward, if you've threatened to harm yourself; it's game over,

You **are** going to the hospital.

There is just no way going to guarantee your patient will be able to make a safe, rational decision for yourself without first being evaluated by a physician in an Emergency Room.

God forbid you accept a refusal from a patient who made suicidal statements, but somehow convinced you they weren't really serious. And then after you leave, your patient goes into the bedroom and kills himself.

Not only would this be an awful burden to bear, but it also potentially opens you up for serious legal action brought against you.

Nope, the risk is just too great. If your patient has said or displayed some sort of suicidal ideation, or attempt, you're going to the hospital.

Likewise, a minor can say they do not want to go to the hospital, but unless there is a parent or guardian that agrees to sign a refusal for them, a minor cannot make that decision for themselves. For this matter I would highly advise you to become familiar with your state laws and local protocols regarding minors, as I've found subtle differences in a lot of different states.

This matter becomes a tad stickier when a child claims they are emancipated.

Again, the laws are varied in several different states regarding who or how a minor can become emancipated. However, in matters of EMS this rarely seems to apply as emancipation is a legal designation and the child would have to furnish some sort of proof of their emancipation. This usually comes in the form of a court document that you can verify. A minor merely telling you they are emancipated isn't usually sufficient.

RESTRAINTS

Details are essential for documenting the specific reasons why you would find yourself needing to physically restrain your patient.

Usually there are just two reasons why you would need to:

1. Your patient has become aggressive or hostile to the point where there is a possibility of physical harm to either themselves or the EMS crew who is attending.

2. Your patient has demonstrated the *potential* for physical violence to the point where the EMS

crew feels a clear threat if they are left unrestrained.

The second reason might present some complications, especially if you document that your patient at the time of transport is not presenting with hostile or violent behavior. However you feel as a medical professional, if you transport this patient unrestrained things might escalate to the point of violence, you should without a doubt restrain your patient. So as you write your chart, one of the focus points needs to be documenting specific details that substantiate your perception of a possible threat.

Did your patient display evidence of violence prior to your arrival?

Are they agitated to the point of hostility?

Are there drugs or alcohol involved?

Has your patient made threats towards you or your partner?

Is your patient in police custody?

Does your patient have a history of violence?

Is your patient displaying bizarre or psychotic tendencies?

All of these are good enough reasons to possibly perceive a threat and want to restrain them. Your job then is to document them so others might also agree with your actions.

Detail the exact reasons why you felt it necessary to restrain your patient and the specific means in which you restrained your patient. It's also probably a good idea to document in your narrative that you assessed your patient's PMS (pulse, motor, sensory) pre and post restraining your patient.

You should be using the minimum amount of force and restraint needed in order to accomplish your goal.

Document the means in which your patient was restrained, i.e. *Staff from fire and EMS crews approached patient with each member securing a limb and easing the patient onto the gurney.*

Also documenting the means used to restrain your patient is extremely important. *Commercial use soft restraints used to secure patient's hands and feet. No signs of pulse, motor or sensory compromise noted before or after patient's restraint.*

Restraining a patient can be either a smooth or messy procedure, depending on the skill level of the EMS providers, the strength and fight the patient wishes to put up and the extraneous factors that might influence the events, such as terrain, weather and lighting.

If any unintended trauma occurred during the process of restraining your patient, this needs to be noted and documented as well. This could apply to both the patient as well as to anyone who helped in the process.

After you have successfully restrained your patient, you should immediately do another rapid assessment to ensure the patient's ABC's have in no way been compromised and their vital signs rechecked.

And of course you are going to need to document this with a timestamp showing the reader there was little to no delay in reassessing your patient after they have been restrained.

Throughout transport you are going to want to do frequent reassessments on your patient. When documenting these vital signs, include a brief note on how your patient current condition, in regards to the restraints. *For example:*

>*...patient appears to have calmed down.*

>*...patient still appears to be extremely agitated.*

...patient continues to show signs of trying to break out of his restraints despite verbal coaching telling him to stop.

>*... patient appears to have fallen asleep.*

Hopefully, the number of times you will be forced to take a patient to the hospital against their will is few and far between. It is a process that can be emotionally wrenching for both patient and provider. When transporting a patient who you have restrained, it's usually a good idea to have someone else in the back of the ambulance to lend another set of eyes to the situation.

If at any point throughout the transport a restrained patient makes an accusation against you, i.e. *they accuse you of stealing from them, assaulting them or in some way mistreating them*, do not confront your patient and escalate the situation. Instead document the patient's exact words and the accusations being leveled against you by the patient.

**Transparency and good documentation will always be your
best defense against false accusations!**

Transporting a Patient against Their Will Example

C: EMS Medic 51 dispatched emergent traffic to a 58 y/o male threatening suicidal ideations (2309). En route to call, dispatch notified EMS that patient apparently has a gun and the scene at this time is not safe. Medic 51 along with Fire Rescue 2 staging at (2314) awaiting clearance to enter by PD.

Scene reported to be secured at (2328). EMS arrived on scene at (2330), noted single family residence which appears clean and well-kept. Arrived at patient's side (2331). Upon our arrival patient found sitting upright on a sofa, approximately 110kg, arms crossed not tracking EMS as we approached. Pt appears awake, however he is refusing to answer questions as he turned his head away upon EMS introductions and if there was anything we could do to help.

Pt's wife found talking to PD, she states that her husband recently lost his job for drinking alcohol on the job and when he came home he became extremely agitated then later deeply depressed. Pt left the house stating he was going to go for a walk and when he came back, he had both alcohol and a gun. According to patient's wife, he started waving this gun in the air telling his wife that he was going to kill himself.

Pt's wife states that he never actually fired the gun, nor pointed it at her or their kids. It was patient's wife who activated 911.

H: According to patient's wife, patient has both a drug and alcohol problem that has been increasingly affecting both his ability to function at work, but also leading to increased tension at home. Wife denies that her husband has displayed any recent acts of violence; however he has made suicidal threats in the past.

Pt also has apparently overdosed multiple times in the past requiring EMS assistance to treat and transport him.

Pt's wife warns EMS that he has stated that he is not going to go "to no fucking hospital" and that he will kill anyone who tries to take him.

Pt apparently also has a past medical history of hypertension and depression, which he is prescribed metoprolol and Prozac. Wife is uncertain about patient's compliance to taking his medications.

Pt has NKDA.

Pt has been home for three hours and has not eaten anything, but has been consuming whiskey. Pt, according to his wife, consumes approximately 2 pints of whiskey a day and does have violent withdrawals when he stops. Pt also has a history of heroin and other opioid abuse.

A: With PD present, patient agreed to allow EMS to take his vital signs. Pt's airway is patent, and he displays no obvious difficulty breathing. Vital signs taken (2342)- Serino P: 99 Strong and regular, B/P 162/98, Resp: 22 Non-Labored, Lung Sounds: Clear and Equal all fields, Skin Warm/Pink/Dry, O2 sat 99% on room air, BGL 132.

Pt has noted odor of possible ETOH coming from his person. Pt admits to drinking "half a bottle" (pint) of Irish whiskey. Pt denies using any illicit narcotics tonight. Pt states that he has not done anything to hurt himself or anyone else and that he would "just like to go to bed."

Pt agrees to a head to toe physical exam (2346) which was found to be unremarkable for any trauma or obvious signs of narcotic use. No obvious track marks on either arm, pt's pupils are both PERRL, respirations are neither slow nor compromised.

Throughout physical exam, patient continues to state that he does not want to go the hospital. Pt does admit to making threats of wanting to hurt himself, but states he states that he wasn't serious.

It is fully explained to patient that it is in his best interest to go with EMS as the behavior he exhibited is a cause for concern for both him and his family.

Pt again states that he is adamant that he is NOT going to the hospital. It is then further explained to the patient, with his wife, PD and fire rescue crew present that based on the nature of his actions, he will be required to go to the hospital and unfortunately at this time he does not have a choice in the matter. He can go with EMS on his own accord, or he will have to be restrained for his safety and ours.

Pt's reply to this is, "Go to hell, I ain't going nowhere." At this time patient attempted to get up and leave the room. He displayed a staggered gait and when EMS and PD attempted to stop him he became aggressive. Pt sat back down on the sofa by PD and told not to move. Pt became increasingly belligerent screaming at EMS and PD to "get the fuck out of my house!"

R: Suicidal Ideation. With PD present, patient's arms were restrained by EMS crew and his feet restrained by fire rescue crew. Pt picked up from sofa and moved to EMS gurney where he was restrained supine with soft restraints securing right hand above his head to gurney frame, left hand to his side and feet restrained to the gurney frame.

Pt's airway and breathing immediately reassessed (2359)- Serino and noted to show no comprise or patient complaint. Pt loaded into ambulance without further incident. Fire Rescue crew member Jake Mares, NRP, rode in with Medic 51 per standard protocols.

T: Transport non emergent at (0002) En route to hospital patient's vital signs reassessed (0004)- Mares. P: 103 Strong/Regular, B/P: 168/100, Resp: 18, non-labored, Skin: W/P/D, O2sat 100% on room air. All four extremities assessed for Pulse/Motor/Sensory deficits distal to the restraints and found to have no compromise. Throughout transport, patient continued to shout obscenities at EMS and made physical threats against us and our families. Pt refused to answer further EMS assessment questions regarding if he was in pain, or if there was anything we could do to make him more comfortable. Radio report called in to hospital (0007)- Serino.
Due to patient being physically restrained and his hostile demeanor, pt was unable to sign the billing form at the end of transport.
Pt brought into ER with hospital security on scene patient transferred to hospital bed, where patient

was restrained. Pt care report taken by Cherith Baker RN (0015).

Chapter 9

Research and Quality Assurance

Our profession is continuously changing. It seems we are constantly receiving updates on everything from protocols to new procedures. Each day someone is coming up with a new and more effective way to help treat our patients.

Up until now you have seen how the PCRs you write can help both the patient and yourself, the provider. But now I want you to see how your PCRs can help the profession as a whole. As you can imagine, EMS depends a great deal on the medical advances achieved through research. However, did you know a tremendous amount of that information used for research, is extrapolated from the very PCRs you write every day?

It's true!

Questions such as:

Which medications seem to have the best results during a cardiac arrest?

Which methods of bagging a patient are most effective?

How do we decide what is really High Quality CPR?

And what are the effects of pushing too much fluid into a patient with hypovolemia secondary to shock?

Have in part been defined or answered using information obtained through EMS patient care reports.

This is why it is so important to be as thorough as possible when it comes to the seemingly endless amounts of drop boxes and data entry that goes into some of the PCRs you create. Each one of those drop boxes can potentially be used to provide your department with either quantitative (based on numbers) or qualitative (written or narrative based) data that your department or service is interested in tracking.

Research is basically a term used to describe the systematic process used to investigate something we want to know more about. Usually the information gathered will then be analyzed against a larger existing body of work in order to gain new insights on pre-existing ideas.

One example of this type of study might be the effectiveness of initiating out-of-hospital therapeutic hypothermia on cardiac arrest patients who EMS has gotten a return of spontaneous circulation (ROSC). Your service might have initiated their own study, or be part of a larger research study that they are taking part in.

Their query might be to find out which process was more beneficial to the patient: to or to not start therapeutic hypothermia.

In order to begin gathering data, they might educate and provide the resources for their ALS units to initiate therapeutic hypothermia on cardiac arrest patients where they have managed to regain ROSC.

They can then analyze the data obtained; possibly comparing it to past circumstances where EMS crews also obtained ROSC but did not initiate hypothermia.

The information obtained from a study such as this might influence future standard of care protocols that could directly change the way our profession treats a particular ailment.

The baseline point of contact information will come from your PCR.

Your willingness to be *complete and thorough* in your charting will help to facilitate gathering necessary information necessary to garner the most complete and accurate results. Even small deviations from what is 100% required to be documented, may skew the results of a research study, resulting in an inaccurate or bias outcome. This is not good for anyone.

No information is better than wrong information!

The benefit of utilizing evidenced based practice is that it helps our patients by eliminating time wasted on ineffectual or inappropriate treatments while also standardizing consistency in the care we provide. This allows a quality of care assurance that we would otherwise not have. Quality Assurance (QA) is a huge part of modern EMS that allows for continuous analysis of how we treat our patients and how we can possibly do it better.

Evidence based practice is also a cost effective way to keep budget costs down by allowing your department to eliminate wasteful products that are no longer relevant.

And as a profession we are constantly modernizing and updating our skills and protocols based on the latest evidence based research. This is part of the reason why first responders are required to take a certain amount of continuing education (CE) hours before they are able to recertify every two years. CEs are great to help solidify what you know and teach you what's new.

And there always seems to be something new! In a relatively short amount of time, EMS has advanced so far from where we first started. So much in fact that, I'll bet a lot of what we are capable of performing out in the field today might seem a bit like science fiction to the first responders of the late 60s and early 70s.

Almost everything about our profession, from where we were to where we are now and where we are going, is based on evidenced based research being gathered and implemented into standard protocol.

By staying engaged about the most current research projects currently being studied, you not only help to remain on the cutting edge of your profession, but also help to stave off feelings of discontentment or burn out.

If your department is not currently doing research, find out when the last time they did do one. Talk with your Quality Assurance (QA) officer or your training department, as they are the ones who are most likely going to be involved in research projects involving your department. You can also read the industry trade magazines, such as JEMS or EMS World that will present current trends in our field as well peer based perspectives from around the nation. In addition, I would also recommend reading the magazine, Prehospital Emergency Care which includes published articles of research and development written by EMS physicians and paramedics.

Another way to stay engaged is to start looking for possible research ideas that you might have in mind. Repetition of calls may spring to light a new and more efficient way to get a patient off scene quicker in the face of a critically traumatic call. Or you might have noticed a similarity in the presentation of COPD patients and you want to investigate the effectiveness of the medications your service carries as opposed to the medications other services might deploy in similar circumstances. Never be afraid to present an idea or question the status quo. EMS is a profession where complacency equates to stagnation. And stagnation is the quickest route to disengagement and mediocracy.

In addition, staying engagement helps to keep you feeling connected to something larger than yourself. Which is something that you are indeed are. You are part of a tremendously noble profession that is predicated on the desire to help strangers in their time of need. Strangers who extend to you a measure of trust that few outside of their family and close friends receive. You are allowed to see them at their worst, no pretense or preparation. These strangers ask for you when they are alone, desperate, hurting and scared. When you become a first responder, you become part of a small brotherhood of men and women who put aside their own personal differences in order to try and bring comfort and hope to someone else. Please don't ever betray that trust. Stay vigilant with those you work with and offer peer-to-peer counseling if you begin to see their morale and valor start to diminish.

Quality Assurance

Nobody is ever perfect. So another benefit of being able to write a strong, detailed PCR is the ability to track a first responder's patterns and consistency. Much like trending a patient's vital signs, looking for improvement or deterioration, a department is also able to follow the clinical and performance trends of their first responders. Usually the responsibility of the Quality Assurance (QA) department, a tremendous amount of their ability to trend comes from the words and details you choose to put into your PCR.

Learning from your mistakes is one of the most effective ways to become a stronger provider. Unfortunately, things often happen so fast in EMS that we might not always be able to reflect on why mistakes occurred or notice your skills in some areas might be starting to wane. Sometimes it might take a second set of eyes reviewing your run reports to be able to see what you cannot.

Most modern ambulance services are continuously auditing and evaluating the PCR's first responders turn in looking for ways to improve areas of adherence to protocols and efficiency of patient care. As we quickly learn in EMS, hindsight is always going to be 20/20. And, if we had the time, I'm sure there isn't one of us who wouldn't look back at a call they ran and think, "*I could have done that better.*"

If only I had known there was a problem, I could have done something about it. Well, perhaps you are not alone in these unnoticed oversights.

Maybe the department as a whole, through a change in procedure, lack of repetitive use or some error in technique is also displaying the same downward shift in performance that you documented in your report.

This is where the QA department can help. By being able to track a run number's times, the clinical skills performed and critical decisions made, a QA officer can begin to look for patterns that might reveal problems in time management, ineffective use of resources or errors in judgement. The QA department can then work towards the goal of identifying specific areas of concern and moving to correct them.

This should be looked at as a tremendous benefit, not a punitive measure. Without the ability to track and evaluate performance measures, EMS as a profession, would run the serious risk of failing to recognize areas of needed improvement and limit future capabilities and potential.

Again, your documentation serves to help not just the patient and the provider, but the profession as a whole.

Usually initiated by the QA Department, these performance measures are broad scope evaluations that encompass everything from the time spent getting dispatched and en route to a call, to the skills, decisions and procedures performed on scene and throughout transport. Everything has the potential to be assessed and everything has the potential to be improved.

And this potential for improvement usually comes in the form of training.

Sometimes the needs for training are limited to you while other times it might be a service wide problem.

For example, say over the course of the first few months this year you continued to document it took you four minutes to get en route to a call but last year at the same time you consistently reported that it only took you two minutes.

What happened? Why suddenly in the span of a year did your time increase by 100%? The QA department might call you in to see if anything had changed. The difference in time might be so subtle that you may never have even noticed the change.

Where were you parking last year as opposed to this year?

Did you have a change in partner?

Are you sleeping well at home?

Did you have a recent call that might have affected you?

Are you responding from a mobile post or are you inside a station?

Do you stay in uniform throughout your shift, or are you having to stop and put your boots on more this year than last?

Are you stepping out of the ambulance to run errands, or parking next to a store that you like to shop at more this year than last?

Sometimes just being made aware of the change in your performance can be enough to get you back to operating at an optimal level with no further training needed to be done. You just simply never noticed a change until someone was able to point it out to you.

Hopefully, adjustments can be made and identified errors corrected.

Likewise, say the department as a whole is reporting first attempt success rates of endotracheal intubation have diminished by over 60% from the previous year. PCR after PCR crews document the need for multiple attempts to successfully intubate their patient.

Of course, any QA officer who notices this would naturally ask themselves why?

How many intubations were attempted last year, compared to this year?

When was the last time our crews had training on advanced airway management?

Do we need to provide more manikins in order for our crews to practice more?

Is this something that looks like it can be corrected, or do protocols need to be changed?

Once an area of concern is discovered, the matter can be presented to the training department in order to coordinate a plan of action.

In a case such as this, it might be beneficial for all ALS personnel to attend a training that reviews technique and practice. If you don't perform a skill on a regular basis, you might have the tendency to let this skill erode. This is why skills that are not often performed, such as delivering a child out in the field, working a pediatric cardiac arrest and performing a cricothyrotomy, should be carefully documented and detailed in your PCR.

NEVER omit or falsify mistakes or poor outcomes because you are afraid of punitive measures. Inefficiencies should be thoroughly documented and evaluated by the QA department in order to see how the procedure went and where there might be room for improvement. Hopefully, any inefficiencies that are documented can be viewed, not as a punishment, but at as a strong resource for future learning.

And learning from our mistakes will always be the most beneficial way our profession will continue to expand and grow.

Chapter 10

Finding the Benefits in Billing

For some reason I've found there almost always seems to be a bit of disconnect between what we do as providers and how that affects our department's ability to get paid. Some first responders believe that our responsibility ends the moment you have turned your patient over to the hospital. How and what the billing department does with my report once it's written, has absolutely nothing to do with how I treat my patient and what I choose to document in my PCR.

Well, I'm here to say nothing can be further from the truth.

One of the most important distinctions you can make as a first responder is to understand you are part of a larger system than just yourself.

You have to understand and appreciate that if your department is doing well, you in a big way, had a hand in that success. And a strong measure of your department's success is their ability to recuperate revenue for the services you provide.

Nearly everything that discussed in this book, from research, training and equipment used to provide the best care for your patients, not to mention the salaries you are paid, is influenced a great deal by the work and tenacity of your billing department. And without a doubt, the most effective resource your billing department has to help them get your department paid is the documentation you provide in your PCR.

So this chapter is here to help you understand how the way in which you choose to document certain information acquired throughout the treatment and care you provide your patient can greatly impact your department's ability to get paid.

So What Happens To Your Report Once You Turn It In?

Because of regulated deadlines and filing requirements, once you submit your PCR it usually will make its first stop in the billing department. If you are submitting your PCR through a computer, as most modern agencies are doing nowadays, your report can be reviewed by numerous departments simultaneously.

Once in the billing department your chart is read and reviewed for a number of things:

- *Are the demographics that might be needed complete?: name, date of birth, social security #, phone number, address.*
- *Is there insurance information?: name of carrier, identification number, billing or customer service phone number.*

- *Does the PCR have a signature?*
- *Are the run times in order?*
- *Is the mileage documented from the scene to the hospital? Typically an EMS system will charge the patient based on the amount of miles they are transported.*

Next the billing department has to figure out two things:

- *How much to charge for the services you rendered.*
- *And: how they are going to get paid.*

Compared to the second part, determining how much the bill is going to be is usually pretty simple. Figuring out how to get it actually paid... *well*, that takes a combination of both tenacity and finesse.

Most EMS services have a standard fee that they charge that is dependent on the level of medical service the patient needed. So, your chart is read for general information that can be quickly extrapolated from your report to determine the level of care you provided for your patient.

- *BLS transport: usually includes treating a patient with most procedures that are non-invasive. Such as providing supplemental oxygen and basic wound care. Typically the least costly type of 911 transport.*
- *ALS 1 transport: usually includes treating a patient with procedures that are typically*

performed by a paramedic, such as initiating an IV, monitoring with a patient with an ECG and performing a 12-lead. This tends to be more expensive than the BLS transport.

- *ALS 2 transport: is usually the most expensive 911 ground transport. It's usually reserved for the most serious of EMS calls and typically involves the use of multiple intravenous medications, advanced airway management, such as endotracheal intubation and cardiac arrest resuscitation.*

Of course there are other services that EMS provides, from interfacility transfers, critical care transports and air ambulance transports; however the costs for these are typically prearranged between the ambulance service and the patient's insurance provider.

So now that we know how much we are going to charge, the billing department has to start looking at how they are going to get reimbursed.

Next a billing specialist will assign a specific International Classification of Diseases (ICD) code, otherwise known as a diagnosis code; to your report based on what you documented was the patient's chief complaint. There are literally thousands of different ICD codes that the billing department must choose from to most accurately fit what you listed as the chief complaint.

For example, the chief complaint listed is abdominal pain: but there are different ICD codes for epigastric pain, lower left abdominal pain, lower right abdominal pain, acute pain... etc.

This is another reason why it is so important to be as specific as possible in your documentation!

Sometimes which ICD code is chosen is also influenced by what you document was your differential diagnosis. Especially if the patient's chief complaint is different from what you state is the differential diagnosis, i.e. patient complains of abdominal pain, but your assessment shows the patient may be experiencing a myocardial infarction.

After assigning a code to your PCR it switches from a clinical document to a financial document and a claim is billed to the patient's private insurance, Medicare, Medicaid or to the patient directly for payment, also known as Self Pay.

Now it becomes a dance of who will pay and who will deny. Remember, the goal of the billing department is to get paid as quickly and as efficiently as possible. The goal of the insurance department is to deny the claim for whatever reason they can, so they don't have to pay.

When an insurance claim is sent back to an EMS service, it takes time and effort to refile and hope that it gets paid on the second or third time around. This is time, money and manpower spent trying to fix something that you could have possibly influenced.

What? How can that be?

Yes it's true! Because what you write has a tremendous influence on whether or not your service can get their claim paid first time through.

And what you need to be aware of is what you can do to help your billing department do their job. Because when they are successful, it's also a huge reflection on how successful you are as both a provider and a professional.

So understand one of the biggest reasons why a claim can be denied is if we do not prove there was an actual medical necessity for transport. We in some way need to show that our patient's medically needed to into the hospital by ambulance.

And before we move any further please understand that I in no way ever want you to lie or "creatively construct facts" in order to accomplish your goal of detailing medical necessity. You can however, present details and select information that can substantiate your goal of proving medical necessity.

Sometimes just being aware of what you are looking for and conscious of needing to in some way prove medical necessity is enough for you to begin documenting details that help build your claim.

For example, if a patient is intoxicated and fell from a standing position, striking his head against a wall, you may begin to start documenting that the patient required ambulance transport due to being unable to drive himself safely and the potential for a severe head injury that could result in further injury up to and including death.

A little extreme? Perhaps. But hopefully you get the point.

I am not creating facts, just presenting them in a way that serves to prove why I felt it is necessary to take my patient into the hospital by ambulance.

In EMS we always hope for the best but prepare for the worst. Well in documentation, especially when it comes to getting your services reimbursed, documenting the potential worst is required.

Another detail that you want to be aware of is to avoid generalities when documenting your patient's condition.

If your patient is bedridden: why are they bedridden?

Are they paralyzed? If so, to what degree are they paralyzed?

If your patient is unable to sign your chart, why are they unable to sign your chart?

Are they unconscious?

Are they refusing to sign?

The billing department will want as much detail as possible that can help them when they file a claim with the insurance department. Anything you can provide to substantiate the reasons why we want to take the patient to the hospital by ambulance will greatly be appreciated.

Another huge detail that will help your billing department to successfully get the claim paid is to have your patient sign your chart. This is an acknowledgement of your patient that they understand there is a financial fee that goes with your services and that they will agree to pay. This also serves as an understanding that they agreed to be transported by 911 ambulance.

If you do not, or are unable to get your patient to sign your chart. Be as specific in your reasons to why this is.

Do they have a medical condition that prevents them from signing? If so, what is it?

Do they show signs of altered mentation? State exactly what is wrong with your patient that is preventing them from signing. And, is this supported in your documentation?

Are they unconscious? Be sure to include why they are unconscious, i.e. Patient unable to sign EMS chart due to being unconscious secondary to multi-system trauma incurred during MVA.

Are they refusing to sign? Why? Are they belligerent? Hostile? Restrained?

Any of these supporting details that will explain why you could not get the patient to sign your chart will help the billing department when making their claim to the insurance agency.

Some interfacility transports require *Medical Necessity* paperwork that needs to be gathered up and taken with the patient. This is an extremely important piece of paperwork as it describes why a physician feels it is necessary for a patient to be transported by an ambulance, rather than by a family member or some other means of transport other than under the care of a medically trained professional. This means that the paperwork you have must be written and signed by a physician in order for it to be reimbursable. This paperwork needs to accompany your PCR when you turn your paperwork in at the end of the day.

Remember, you and the billing department are ultimately on the same team. Sometimes I tend to think of it in terms of a football team. The offense will always need the defense to do their part in order to win a game. No single player can accomplish the team's goal; it requires an understanding and cooperation of everyone involved to accomplish the task at hand. The same is true in EMS. Without the work and carefully crafted documentation provided by the first responders, the billing department wouldn't be able to get the department paid. Without the billing department, first responders would be paid less, working with less than the adequate equipment, or perhaps even laid off and unemployed. It's a symbiotic relationship that keeps us all employed and serving the community we live in.

Chapter 11

Abdominal Calls

Upon Our Arrival:

- How the patient was found (*ambulatory/curled up on ground knees flexed*)?
- Patient's mentation?
- Is there any unusual or unpleasant odors you can detect or find evidence of (*feces/vomit*)?
- Is there anything on scene that seems to be excessively out of the ordinary (*beer cans, pizza boxes, littered trash, etc.*)?

History:

- How long have they been in pain?
- Can they describe it (*crampy/sharp/burning*)?
- Is this a female of child bearing age, last menstrual cycle, are they sexually active (*ectopic pregnancy*)?
- Last bowel movement? Did it appear normal (*color/diarrhea*)? Was there any blood noted or was it darker and more tar like than usual (*possible GI Bleed*)?
- Have they vomited since they began having this pain?
- Have they ever had this pain before?
- Has anything changed in their diet recently?

- Any unexpected or unusual weight loss or gain?
- Is anyone else in the household experiencing similar pain (*food poisoning/toxicity*)?
- Do they still have all of their internal organs, or have any been surgically removed?
- Have they recently experienced any trauma to the abdomen (*assault/fall/sports injury*)?
- Any cardiac history (*MI, AAA*)?

Medications:

- Any medications that can lead you to forming a differential diagnosis?
- Are they compliant with all meds?
- Do they take any over the counter meds?

Social:

- Do they abuse recreational drugs?
- Are they an alcoholic?

Physical Assessment:

- Which quadrant does it hurt (*RUQ, LUQ, RLQ, LLQ*)?
- Patient's skin color. Any signs of shock, internal hemorrhage or liver dysfunction?
- Visualization of abdomen: any signs of ecchymosis or discoloration?
- Palpation of abdomen: any masses, pulsations, rigidity or distention noted?

Chapter 12

Acute Coronary Syndrome

Upon our arrival:

- Note for scene safety

History:

- Ascertain duration of chest pain.
- What was patient doing at time of onset (*exertional vs. non-exertional*)?
- What symptoms did patient present with (*chest pain, shortness of breath, nausea, vomiting, syncope*)?
- Did the patient do anything to try and treat this discomfort (*antacids, aspirin, nitroglycerin, rest*) and did it work?
- Has the patient ever had this type of discomfort before?
- Does the patient have a significant cardiac history?
- Any recent life changes in patient's history (*loss of a job, death of a spouse/child, divorce*)?
- **Risk factors**: (*sedentary life style, obesity, high cholesterol, social risks: smoking, drinking*).
- Any recent trauma to the chest (*MVA, falls, assault*)?

- Any recent bouts of violent coughing (*flu, emphysema, bronchitis*)?
- Does the patient have a family history of cardiac problems?

Medications:

- Does patient take any cardiac medications prescribed by a doctor (*Digoxin, Nitroglycerin, Atenolol*)?
- Does patient take any preventative measures (*regular doctor visits, daily exercise, aspirin a day*)
- Are they compliant with all medications?
- Are the medications the patient takes still within the expiration date?
- Where does patient store his medications (*Nitro loses potency if exposed to light*)?

Social:

- Smoker? How many cigarettes per day and for how long have they been smoking (*days, months, years?*).
- Alcohol user? How often do they drink (*every day, social, hardly ever*) and do they have problems when they stop drinking (DT, tremors, seizures)?
- Do they take illicit or recreational drugs? What kind and how often. Do they take narcotics that could increase the demand of oxygen for the heart (*cocaine, methamphetamines*)?

Physical Assessment:

- What is patient's level of consciousness (*awake and oriented, anxious, sense of impending doom, confusion*)?
- How they appear (*skin color, diaphoresis, labored breathing, vomiting*).
- As specific as you can, where the pain is located (*substernal, left pectoral region, subclavian region*).
- Does the pain radiate anywhere? Again, be as specific as possible.
- Without leading your patient, try to use their own words to describe the pain (*sharp, crampy, burning, dull*).
- How do you interpret the cardiac monitor's initial rhythm?
- Note time and who performed the first 12 lead and your interpretation of it.
- Note times, routes and dosages of all medications administered and who administered them.
- If you need to contact medical control, note time, who physician was and the specific orders they gave you.

Chapter 13

Altered Mentation

Upon Our Arrival:

- Scene survey: note anything that stands out as a possible cause for patient condition (*drug paraphernalia, empty medication vials, alcohol, signs of violence*).
- Provide a specific detailing of your patient's mental condition based on the AVPU scale (*are they tracking you, are they awake, are they oriented some things, but not others? If so then to what*).
- Is there evidence of gross hemorrhaging?
- Are there any witnesses that can provide information? If so, document who they are and what relation they are to the patient (*wife, friend, by-stander*).
- Note position patient was found and where (*supine on the floor, prone on the grass, near a pool, slumped over on his left side in a recliner*).
- Is there a "Vial of Life" or Medication List discovered on scene?

History:

- Medical history that lends itself to explaining current situation (*seizure, diabetic, dementia, substance abuse*).

- Does anyone know how long the patient has been in this condition?
- Is this an acute problem or chronic?
- Was the patient complaining of anything out of the ordinary or recently acting bizarre (*terrible headache, visual disturbances, gradual or sudden onset of irritability or irrationality*)?
- Has a similar situation happened before in the past? If so, then when? What was diagnosed and how was it treated?
- Any recent history of depression?
- Sudden life changes (*divorce, death of a loved one, loss of a job*)?
- Recent physical trauma within the last few days (*assault, fall*)?
- Any recent complaints of vertigo, dizziness, or loss of balance?

Medications:

- Does patient take any medications that might help you make a differential diagnosis (*hypertension, diabetes, seizure, dementia*)?
- Is patient compliant with taking their prescribed medications?
- Are there any recent prescription changes or increase/decrease in dosages?

Social:

- Does patient take illicit or recreational drugs?
- Is patient a chronic ETOH user?

Physical Assessment:

- If patient has altered mentation note your full head to toe exam looking for any signs of DCAP-BTLS (*especially take note to document how the patient's pupils presented: blown/constricted/unequal, if there is any signs of oral trauma: tongue bitten after possible seizure and if possible, patient's speech pattern: slurred/dysphasia/aphasia*).
- What is the patient's respiration pattern (*Kussmaul, Cheyne-Stokes, Biot's, Ataxic, Bradypnea*)?
- Is patient able to provide any symptoms that might help lead you to a differential diagnosis (*nausea, headache, visual disturbances*)?
- Any physical signs of possible drug abuse (*needle marks: fresh/old*)
- Are there any medical bracelets, necklaces?
- What is the patient's blood glucose level?
- Are there any signs of incontinence?

Chapter 14

Cardiac Arrest

Upon our arrival:

- Was this a witnessed arrest? If so, what time did patient lose a pulse? Did the patient say or complain of anything prior to losing consciousness?
- Does this appear to be a medical or trauma arrest?
- How and where is the patient positioned and have they been moved by anyone?
- Has CPR been started by anyone prior to EMS arrival and if so, who and for how long? Did they have an automated external defibrillator available to them and was a shock deployed prior to EMS arrival?
- Is there any drug paraphernalia in plain view near the patient?
- Is there a weapon on scene (*suicide*)?
- Is there any sign of a suicide note?

History:

- Does the patient have a cardiac history (*CAD, MI, CHF, Cardiogenic Shock*) including cardiac surgeries (*CABG*)? If so has patient previously suffered a cardiac arrest?

Medications:

- Does the patient take any prescription medications that indicate a past cardiac history (*NTG, beta blockers, diuretics*)?
- Has the patient been compliant with these medications?

Social:

- Does the patient have a history of substance abuse (*cocaine/methamphetamines or heroin/opioids*)?
- Has the patient overdosed in the past?
- Is the patient an alcoholic?

Physical Assessment:

- What is initial cardiac rhythm (*asystole, v-fib, PEA*)?
- Did patient need to be moved to accommodate EMS resuscitation efforts?
- Time CPR started by EMS and by whom.
- Signs of vomit or blood in airway?
- Note how airway was managed (*OPA, extraglottic airway, ET intubation*).
- Any obvious signs of trauma noted?
- Note the 5 H's and T's and document each with explanation of any relevant findings.

- Any sign of a cardiac surgical scar noted upon patient's chest.
- Did patient's chest require the need to be shaved prior to defibrillation pads?
- What time was first shock administered and at what Joule setting.
- Time IV was established, what gage and where it was placed.
- Note IV fluid and amount administered.
- Note with a timestamp all ACLS interventions and who administered them (*Epi, Shock, Amiodarone, Shock, etc...*).
- Note capnography readings.
- If return of spontaneous circulation is achieved, note the time, capnography quantitative figure and cardiac rhythm.
- Note how patient was moved from ground to gurney.
- Note baseline vital signs as soon as you can and q. five minutes throughout transport.

Chapter 15

Cerebral Vascular Accidents

Upon our arrival:

- Note position patient found and if they happen to be tracking you upon arrival.
- Any witnesses that can provide a credible time of onset for patient's signs and symptoms?

History:

- Does patient have a previous history of hypertension?
- Any cardiac history, specifically a-fib.
- Does the patient smoke cigarettes? If so how much and for how long have they done so?
- Any recent history of long plane or car trips that required the patient to be sedentary for an extended period of time?
- Is the patient pregnant?
- Does the patient have a history of diabetes?
- Has the patient recently had a long bone fracture or some other form of surgery?
- Has the patient recently been involved in a traumatic incident (*assault, fall, MVA, head injury*)?

- Has the patient recently been complaining of a headache or visual disturbances?
- Has the patient ever suffered a stroke or stroke-like symptoms that resolved itself within the last few weeks?
- Has patient recently been complaining of feelings of vertigo, loss of balance or nausea?
- Does the patient have a history of blood clotting disorders, DVT's or hypercoagulation?
- Any recent history of syncope?

Medications:

- Does the patient take hypertensive medications (*Metoprolol, Atenolol Carvedilol*) ?
- Does the patient take anticoagulation medication (*Plavix, Lovenox, Coumadin*)?
- Is the patient taking oral birth control pills?
- Any diabetic medications?
- Is patient

Social:

- Note any substance abuse issues, especially those that might raise the patient's blood pressure such as cocaine and methamphetamines.

Physical Assessment:

- Note patient's current level of consciousness (*LOC*).

- Any obvious physical or mental impairments (*aphasia, hemiparesis*).
- Perform a standard FAST or Cincinnati Stroke Scale test and note the findings and time performed.
- Obtain a BGL!
- Try to narrow down the time of symptom onset and note how you were able to come to that time (*Pt's wife states she believes her husband's mentation began to drop at 11 pm, because they were watching the evening news when she noticed he had slightly slurred speech and an obvious left sided facial droop*).
- Depending on local protocol: notify your destination hospital as early as possible and call a Stroke Alert.
- Begin trending vital signs, noting time and changes in patient's mentation and physical disabilities.

Chapter 16

Geriatric Calls

Upon Our Arrival:

- Consider the need for additional resources early on.
- Take special note of where the scene is (patient's house, stranger's house, supermarket, car or on the side of the road) don't just write "residential house," if that's the case, then who's house is it?
- Is this a medical call or trauma? Or both?

History:

- Is this a chronic situation (*dementia*) or an acute problem (*delirium, CVA, hypoglycemia*)?
- Is there a history of violence or aggression?
- History of depression or suicidal ideation?
- Always keep an eye out for possible signs of elder abuse (*afraid to speak, signs of bruising or swelling, adult children not allowing you to examine the patient thoroughly*). If you do suspect, do not confront person you suspect as an abuser, document and notify police/hospital.
- Fully examine co-morbidities and find out if there are any recent changes or diagnoses that might help you decide on a differential diagnosis.
- Does patient live alone, with children or at an assisted living/nursing home?

- How is the house maintained (*proper heating/air conditioning depending on weather, house clean or cluttered and dirty, is their proper food in the refrigerator and cabinets or does the patient appear to be going without proper nutrition*).
- Any recent lifestyle changes (*divorce, death of a spouse/child, recently received a poor medical diagnosis*)

Medications:

- Who is in charge of the patient's medications? Who dispenses the medications and ensures they are taken correctly or is the patient in charge of managing their medications?
- Does the patient appear to be capable of managing their own medications (*do meds appear organized, are they in prescription vials or are they out and thrown together in a mixed bag*)
- Are patient's medications in child protective vials? If so, is patient still able to open them up?
- Does patient know which medications they are on? Do they know when they are supposed to take them and why they are prescribed?
- Do medications appear to be from same physician or are their various prescriptions of the same medication filled by several physicians?
- Are medications still in date or have they expired?

- Do medications appear to be missing (*accidental/intentional overdose, especially narcotic pain killers*)?

Social:

- Note any signs of alcohol or drug abuse.
- Does patient smoke cigarettes, how many and for how long.
- Does patient appear to have any social interactions with other people (*family, friends or are they isolated*)?

Physical Assessment:

- What is patient's level of consciousness? Is this normal for them or is this something new?
- Any signs of trauma (*new/older, one spot or diffuse and in various states of healing*)?
- Is patient hostile or aggressive?
- Does patient appear to be able to take care of themselves (*malnourished, unkempt, house in a state of disrepair*)
- Get a BGL and perform a CVA exam.
- If patient lives alone, are they ambulatory?

Chapter 17

Non Traumatic Hemorrhage

Upon our arrival:

- Note any obvious signs of blood (*on the floor, in the bathroom, in the toilet*)

History:

- Is this a new onset of bleeding or is this something that the patient has been forced to deal with before?
- Is this obvious blood in the patient's stool (*bright red blood, melena*)?
- Does the patient have a history of ulcers or gastrointestinal problems?
- Does patient have any history of hemorrhoids or cancer?
- When was the last time they had a normal bowel movement?
- Is this an uncontrollable nose bleed (*epistaxis*)? How long have they been bleeding from the nose? What caused it to start bleeding (*trauma, recent surgery, drug use*)?
- Is this uncontrollable bleeding from the vaginal area?
- How long have they been bleeding?

- How many sanitary napkins have they gone through?
- Was there any clumping or obvious tissue material in the bleeding?
- Has your patient ever had this type of problem before?
- Could they possibly be pregnant?
- Are they sexually active?
- Any pain upon urination or foul odor (*STD*)?
- Are they suffering any pain with this bleeding?
- Has your patient recently been out of the country?
- Are they coughing or vomiting blood? Is it frank red blood or does it have the appearance of coffee grounds.
- Do they have a history of alcoholism or hypertension (*esophageal varices*)?

Medications:

- Is the patient on any blood thinners (*Plavix, Coumadin*)?

Social:

- Is your patient a chronic alcoholic?
- Does your patient inhale (*snort*) narcotics through the nasal passages?

Physical Assessment:

- What is your patient's mentation upon your arrival?

- What is their skin color, temperature and condition (*pink vs pale, warm vs cool/cold, dry vs clammy/diaphoretic*).
- How is your patient's pulse (*weak, thready, regular, irregular*)?
- If patient presents with signs of hypovolemic shock (*low B/P, tachycardia, cool/clammy skin*) document rapid transport and your interventions for shock management (*IV fluids, supplemental oxygen, heat up your ambulance, warm blankets*)
- Document all interventions with a time stamp and who initiated them.

Chapter 18

OB/Gyn Calls

Upon our arrival:

- Take note of time of day, location and the possibility that you may be dealing with an imminent delivery.

History:

- Does patient know if they are possibly pregnant or not (*last menstrual cycle, sexually active*)?
- Is there any abdominal pain (*ask patient to describe the pain and origin, and severity of the pain, ask if she's had this pain before in the past, and try to r/o as many causes that you are able to: appendicitis, ovarian cysts, endometriosis, UTI, STD, and ectopic pregnancy*)?
- Has there been any vaginal discharge or bleeding (*spotting, frank red blood, number of pads she has gone through and how fast*)?
- Has patient had any recent bouts of syncope, nausea/vomiting or any loose stools with blood?
- Find out if there has been any discoloration with her urine or any unusually foul smells that she's noticed from her vagina (*bacterial vaginosis, UTI, STD*).

- Any surgical procedures that would make it impossible for your patient to be pregnant (*hysterectomy, tubal ligation*)?
- If pregnant, does patient know her due date?
- Is she being seen by a physician for pre-natal care? Any unusual occurrences that she is aware of (*twins, breech, possible physical deformities*)?
- Has patient had any problems with any of her pregnancies before in the past (*C-sections, low birth weight, spontaneous abortions, miscarriages*)?
- Find out the Para/Gravida for this pregnancy.
- Has your patient been treated for gestational diabetes?
- Is she under any doctor's orders for bed rest?
- Concerns for pre/eclampsia (*recent swelling of feet, hands, or headaches/visual disturbances*)?
- When did her water break?
- Any contractions (*how far apart and how severe*)?
- Based on medical history, is this a high risk pregnancy.

Medications:

- Is patient taking oral contraception (*birth control pills*)?
- Has patient been taking any medications to manage abdominal/pelvic pain?
- Find out if patient has missed any days of her medication.

Social:

- Does patient smoke cigarettes? Has she continued to do so throughout pregnancy (*increased risk for high risk pregnancy*)?
- Does your patient drink alcohol (*increased risk of pregnancy*)?
- Any illicit drug use before or during pregnancy? Is she going to possibly need the use of naloxone? Remember, if mother is going through withdrawals, so is the fetus.

Physical Assessment:

- What is patient's mentation upon arrival (*is she tracking you, does she know why you are there, who activated 911*)?
- Skin color (*does patient appear to be in shock from blood loss*)?
- Any noted edema in feet or hands?
- Is patient's blood pressure higher than normal?
- What is patient's BGL?
- Where does it hurt? Palpate from area farthest away and move work your way towards the pain (*feeling the abdomen for any masses, pulsations, tenderness, rigidity, discoloration*).
- Is delivery imminent (*crowning, limb/cord/breech presentation*)?
- If you are required to deliver baby, document the PPE that you put on, time that you started, the

presentation of the baby and the APGAR score at 1 and 5 minutes.

Chapter 19

Overdose/Poisoning

Upon our arrival:

- Make note of any potential safety concerns and need for additional assistance *(police, fire, additional EMS)*.
- If necessary, note the location and time you staged waiting for scene to become secure.
- Once on scene, make a note of the scene *(residential, single story house, a car in a parking lot, the beach)*.
- Take note of anything that might give you an idea of what the patient may have been poisoned with.
- Is the patient a child who may have swallowed house products or parent's medications?
- Note any obvious drug paraphernalia or evidence of a crime *(syringes, needles, knives, gun, ampules and narcotics in plain sight: however without knowing for certain what it is, document it as "substance that looks like it might be marijuana" or "white powder left on table that has the appearance of a narcotic such as heroin or cocaine.")*.

- Note any signs of violence (*broken furniture, broken windows, possible bullet holes in the walls, blood on the floor*).
- Scan scene for any possible indications that this might be a suicide attempt (*suicide note*). If found, document it.
- Take care not to disturb a potential crime scene.

History:

- Attempt to ascertain if this was an accidental or intentional overdose or poisoning.
- Does patient have a history of substance abuse?
- Has patient in the past overdosed? Have they required EMS to resuscitate them?
- When was the patient last seen at their baseline mentation?
- Does the patient have a psychiatric history? Are they on tricyclic antidepressants?
- Does your patient's history include suicide attempts or ideations?
- Any recent lifestyle changes (*divorce, death of a spouse or child, loss of a job*)?
- Does your patient go in for dialysis? Have they missed any of their scheduled appointments?
- What does patient do for a living and could they have been exposed to something toxic at their place of employment (*organophosphate pesticides, heavy metals, carbon monoxide, radiation*)?

- If event happens at the patient's place of employment, be sure to ask for any materials safety data sheets that could possibly be involved.

Medications:

- Does your patient take psychiatric medication?
- Any pain killers or narcotic analgesics?
- Does the amount of pills in the vial seem to match the intended dosage?

Social:

- Does patient have any history of substance abuse?
- Is patient a chronic alcoholic?

Physical Assessment:

- What is your patient's mentation at time of assessment (*alert and conscious, verbal, painful, unresponsive*)?
- Is their airway patent (*vomit, frothing at the mouth*)? Is it expected to stay patent (*diminishing LOC, hoarse speech, excessive drooling, blood or vomiting*)?
- Breathing (*Rate depth and quality, is this someone who you are going to have to immediately manage their airway. Document your reasons.*)
- Circulation (*fast, slow, weak, irregular, bounding*)
- Skin condition (*does your patient feel hot, dry, poor turgor, track marks on arms or feet*).

- Eyes (*are the pupils equal and reactive to light pinpoint constricted, dilated, unequal*).
- Cardiac monitor (*tachycardia, bradycardia, wide QRS, sine wave, peaked T waves*)
- Is patient acting bizarre or belligerent?
- Do you anticipate needing to restrain your patient, if so why?

Chapter 20

Respiratory Emergencies

Upon our arrival:

- Note the presence of anything that may be indicative of a chronic respiratory problem (*ashtrays filled with cigarette butts, the strong smell of cigarettes throughout the patient's residence, oxygen tubing stretched on the ground, oxygen tanks, metered dose inhalers*)

History:

- Based on the patient's past medical history, is this an acute or chronic problem (*pneumonia, choking/toxins/pulmonary embolism/respiratory infection vs. COPD/CHF/Tuberculosis*)?
- Does the patient have a medical history that includes respiratory problems (*asthma, emphysema, chronic bronchitis, lung cancer, spontaneous pneumothorax*)?
- Has patient had a productive cough? If so, document the color and consistency (*pinkish sputum-CHF/pulmonary embolism/TB, greenish mucus- pneumonia, respiratory infection, chronic bronchitis*).
- What was patient doing at the time of dyspnea (*exertional vs non-exertional onset*)?

- Is patient able to sleep lying flat, or do they require the use of pillows in order to keep them propped up (*nocturnal dyspnea*)?
- Does patient use a CPAP machine?
- Has patient been feeling more tired than usual?
- Did patient lose consciousness?
- Has patient been involved in any recent traumatic events (*MVA/assault/falls*)?
- Has the patient recently had surgery (*PE*)?
- Does the patient have any cardiac history (*A-Fib, AV heart blocks, runs of V-Tach*)?
- Does patient ever get short of breath for no apparent reason (*CHF/COPD*)?
- Is patient allergic to anything or have they been exposed to a possible allergen?
- Has patient recently had any unusual weight gains or losses (*cancer/CHF*)?
- Does patient have any recent flu-like symptoms (*influenza, H1N1, Coronavirus 19*).
- Is patient morbidly obese (*size of stomach preventing full expansion of the diaphragm leading to increasing dyspnea*)?

Medications:

- Does patient have any medications indicative of chronic respiratory problems (*oxygen, albuterol, Atrovent, corticosteroids*)?
- Does patient take medications for cardiac problems that might also have respiratory issues

(*beta-blockers, calcium channel blockers, diuretics, anticoagulants*)?

- Is patient compliant with their medications?

Social:

- Does patient smoke cigarettes? If so, how many and for how long (*# of packs x # of years*)?
- Does patient work in a field that may contain elements harmful to their lungs (*firefighter, coal mine, construction, industrial plant*)?

Physical Assessment:

- What is patient's mentation upon your arrival (*awake and oriented, somnolent, stuporous, signs of hypoxic rage, irritability, restlessness, unconscious, unresponsive*)?
- Respiratory rate, rhythm and quality (*tachypnea, bradypnea, irregular, Kussmaul, Cheyne's Stokes, Biot's, Ataxic*)
- Lung Sounds (*clear and equal bilaterally, diminished, crackles, rales, rhonchi, absent*)?
- Normal chest expansion with each respiration?
- Palpate the intercostal muscles as patient takes a deep breath, feel for crepitus, paradoxical movement and inability to take a deep breath due to pain.
- Skin Color (*pale, cyanotic, flushed, cherry red*)
- O2 saturation (*room air vs with supplemental oxygen*)

- Capnography: normal wave with plateau, shark fin (*COPD/Asthma*), large wave short plateau (*bradypnea/hypercarbia*), small fast waves (*tachypnea/hypocarbia*).
- Place patient on cardiac monitor, including 12 lead and document the results.
- Note IV site, # of attempts/success, catheter gage and fluid.
- Document time, reason and effect of each medication administered.
- Look for edema in the feet and hands.
- Inspect fingers for signs of clubbing (*COPD*).
- Note the presence of a barrel shaped chest.
- Is the patient required to breath using accessory muscles or through pursed lips?
- Document supplemental oxygen delivery (*nasal cannula, non-rebreather mask, CPAP, Bag Valve Mask*).
- Document awareness of hypoxic drive when administering supplemental oxygen to patients who have a history of COPD. If patient begins to slow their breathing or becomes apneic provide positive pressure ventilation via a bag valve mask and document the incident.
- Make note of the position you placed patient in for transport.

Chapter 21

Sick Calls

Upon our arrival:

- Document scene safety and the presence of anything out of the ordinary (*cluttered house, stockpiled alcohol cans/bottles, animal feces, odor of animal urine, insect activity*).

History:

- How long as patient been feeling sick?
- What symptoms is the patient complaining of (*nausea/vomiting, headache/vertigo*)?
- Is this anything they have had before?
- Is anyone else in the home complaining of similar symptoms?
- Has anyone been recently ill?
- Does anything the patient has done, prior to EMS activation, make them feel better (*antacids, aspirin, rest*)?
- Is their illness causing them any pain?
- Have there been any signs of delirium or altered mentation?
- Is the patient bedridden or confined to a wheelchair (*decubitus ulcer, Foley Catheter, other areas of possible infection or sepsis*)?

- Any recent changes in diet, medications or lifestyle (*new job, loss of job, stressful situations: loss of spouse/child*).
- Are there any signs of failure to thrive (*house in state of disrepair, dirty or soiled bedsheets that the patient is laying on, emaciated appearance*)?
- Any changes in bowel movements (*odor, consistency, frequency, solid/watery*).
- Any recent weakness or inability to ambulate?
- Any unusual odors or pain when urinating?
- Any chronic problems that may have deteriorated to cause these symptoms (*poorly managed diabetes, hypertension, liver or kidney problems, cancer*)?
- Any sudden changes in weight loss or gain?
- Is there any chance your patient is pregnant (*morning sickness, last menstrual cycle, sexually active, STD's*)?
- Is your patient a pediatric (*RSV, Influenza, chicken pox, measles*)?

Medications:

- Has your patient been compliant with all mediations they are currently prescribed?
- Who handles the patient's medications (*any chance of dementia, poor organization, possibility of meds being forgotten or taken more than they should*)?

- Any new or recent medications that could be having an adverse effect when taken with other medications?
- Does your patient take antidepressants or other psychiatric medications?

Social:

- Is your patient an alcoholic? Do they suffer from withdrawals when they stop drinking alcohol?
- Is your patient a chronic drug abuser? Do they suffer withdrawals when they stop using?
- Has your patient ever been diagnosed as clinically depressed?

Physical Assessment:

- What is your patient's level of consciousness (*alert and oriented/delirious/unconscious*)?
- Is airway currently patent and is it expected to stay that way (*decreased mentation, vomiting, somnolent*)?
- Does patient appear to be dehydrated (*vomiting, diarrhea*)?
- Skin color, temperature (*signs of hypovolemic or septic shock*)?
- Is patient able to describe symptoms to you and do they match the signs that you are seeing?
- Are there any obvious routes of possible infection that you can see (*ulcerations, dark urine with sediment in Foley bag, cellulitis, open wounds with pus and foul odors*)?

- If necessary and applicable to your local protocols, activate a sepsis alert early and provide rapid transport.

Chapter 22

Animal Bites and Stings

Upon our arrival:

- Ensure you document the need for any additional resources that might be needed to secure the scene.
- If staging is necessary, document where you stage and the time you arrive on scene.

History:

- Document what the nature of injury is (*dog bite, insect stings, snake bite*).
- Explore any known allergies the patient may lead to possible anaphylaxis.
- Note the time that the event occurred.
- Was there a loss of consciousness?
- Has the animal/insect that caused the damage been captured?
- If this is a domestic animal, is there an owner on scene who can provide shot records and medical history?

Social: N/A

Medications:

- Does patient have an EpiPen?
- Was an Epi Pen used prior to your arrival?
- Was patient given diphenhydramine (Benadryl) prior to EMS arrival?

Physical Examination:

- What is the patient's level of consciousness (awake and oriented, disoriented, unconscious)?
- Is the airway patent and is it expected to remain patent (signs of tongue swelling up, laryngeal edema, hoarse voice)?
- How is the patient's current state of breathing (labored, shallow, tachypnea, bradypnea)?
- Document lung sounds.
- If this is an isolated injury focus your assessment to the care and management of the wound.
- If there is a possibility for anaphylaxis, note the state of the patient's skin (hives, uticaria, wheals)?
- If the wound is suspected to be caused by a venomous animal (snake, spider, scorpion) visualize the area of the wound and use a pen to outline the current area of irritation and redness. Upon reassessment see if the area has spread outside of your initial outline. Document the spread and the speed in which it appears to be spreading.

- If practical and safe, bring any snake, insect or spider to the hospital for identification and assistance for treatment.
- In your documentation DO NOT guess what type/breed you believe the animal that caused damage to be. You can document the size, color and provide a brief description of the animal/insect. You can speculate as to what it might be, i.e. *The spider was possibly a black widow due to it's shiny black appearance, with a large black abdominal segment that featured a red hour glass shape.*
- Document the time and outcome for any interventions you provide, including airway management, if necessary, supplemental oxygen, IV administration of medications (*epinephrine, diphenhydramine*).

Chapter 23

Assaults

Upon our arrival:

- Document the need for possible scene safety.
- If you are required to stage while, waiting for the scene to become safe, be sure to document both the time you stage and the time you actually arrive on scene.
- Once on scene, document any obvious signs of traumatic events that could involve your patient (*shattered windows, smashed furniture, broken glass, a weapon, any signs of blood: pools or streaks on the walls*).
- Document who was the first on scene to initiate medical care (*police, first responders, by-standards, family*): note the person or service that initiated care and what it was that they did.
- How many patients do you have on scene? Note the need for additional resources and if you had to declare yourself the incident commander of a multi-casualty event.

History:

- Are there any bystanders that can give you an idea of what happened (*remember that anything a bystander happens to tell you is subjective and may not be the most reliable of information: always attribute the information obtained to the source from which you received it.*)

- Does this appear to be a sexual assault (*if so, remember you are dealing with a very delicate crime scene: try not to destroy potential evidence: clothing, potential DNA: more than likely your chart will be subpoenaed, so be sure to document as many details as you can.*)? If you have local protocols for activating a Sexual Assault Nursing Examiner (SANE) do so and document it.

- Are there any weapons on scene that can help you determine what was used in the assault (*bloody pipe, broken beer bottle, knife*)?

- Is your patient an infant, pediatric, adult with limited mental capacities or a geriatric? Each of these circumstances needs to be documented and reported to police if they are not already on scene. One of the highest responsibilities we have as first responders is to always be an advocate for our patients. This becomes especially true if our patient is in a position where they cannot or have limited ability to advocate for themselves.

Medications:

- Does patient take any medications that tend to be abused (*pain killers, narcotics*)? Does patient have problems when he stops taking his medications (*tremors, withdrawals*)?

Social:

- Is there evidence of drug or alcohol use that precipitated the assault?
- Could mask pain and be a contributing factor to the situation.
- Does your patient appear to be intoxicated or under the influence of narcotics (*slurred words, odor of ETOH on their breath, pinpoint pupils*)?

Physical Assessment:

- Is there any obvious life threatening hemorrhage that you see upon arrival at your patient?
- What is patient's level of consciousness (*are they tracking you upon approach, disoriented, in a stupor, responsive only to verbal stimulus, unconscious*)?
- Does your patient have a patent airway upon your arrival, or do they have an injury that might be expected to affect it (*head injury affecting LOC, trauma to naso/oral pharynx, blunt or penetrating trauma to the neck, signs of a sucking chest wound*)
- Document a thorough head to toe physical assessment
- If getting patient trauma naked, note how you preserved modesty with a sheet or blanket and document how you carefully handled their

clothing (*again this is all possibly vital evidence involved in a crime scene*). When cutting clothes off, do not cut through gunshot wounds, knife penetration sites and place these clothes ideally in a paper bag, or a biohazard bag.

- Does the patient appear to be in shock? If so treat for that, with warm blanket, turning the temperature up in the ambulance, IV fluids.
- Any signs of a depressed skull fracture?
- Any Battle's signs or "raccoon eyes?"
- Is there any sign of drainage (*blood, CSF*) from the ears?
- Is the bridge of the nose intact? How about the teeth, any appear to be recently knocked loose? Ask the patient to use their tongue to see if any teach are loose.
- Neck pain upon palpation, or is there any signs of jugular vein distention (JVD), tracheal deviation?
- Clavicles stable? Intercostal muscles intact? Have the patient take a deep breath with your hands on their ribs: is there any instability, crepitus, paradoxical movement, pain?
- Palpate the abdomen, all four quadrants: any discoloration, rigidity, tenderness, lacerations or punctures?
- Pelvis stable? If there are signs of neurological impairment: assess male patients for the presence of priapism.
- Inspect all four extremities for any deformities, swellings and lacerations: mostly checking for

PMS: pulse, motor (*can they wiggle their toes/fingers upon command*) and sensation (*can they tell which foot/hand you are touching*).

- Inspect the posterior prior to putting patient on backboard (*you may not get another chance to inspect this area*).

Chapter 24

Burns

Upon our arrival:

- Document if the scene location is an open or closed area.
- Is the scene safe for you to enter?
- Is there any possibility that you might need additional resources that have further training or SCBA to enter scene.
- Any possibility of smoke exposure (*remember the pulse oximetry reading might not be 100% accurate if the patient was exposed to high levels of carbon monoxide*).
- What type of burn is it you are dealing with (*thermal, electrical, radiation, chemical*)?
- Was there an explosion (*primary, secondary, tertiary injuries*)?
- Is there other trauma involved then in addition to the burn?
- Was patient knocked unconscious?
- What time did the incident happen? Is this something that just happened, or is this something that the patient has been trying to treat on their own for some time (*site infected, gangrenous*)?
- How long was the patient exposed to the material that caused the burn?

History:

- Was there a medical incident that preceded the burn (*hypoglycemia, syncope, cardiac arrest*)?
- Was there any treatment provided prior to EMS arrival? If so, by whom and what did they do (*bandage, extricate, mouth to mouth, resuscitation*)?

Medications:

- Is the patient taking any medications that might mask normal pain or shock response in their vital signs (*beta blockers, analgesics*)

Social:

- Is the patient taking any illicit narcotics that might mask pain response to vital signs (*opioids, stimulants, hallucinogens*).

Physical Assessment:

- Are there any signs of airway involvement (*soot in the nose, hoarse throat, difficulty breathing*)?
- Is this someone that is going to possibly require rapid sequence intubation (RSI)?
- What is the status of the patient's clothing and did they need to be removed quickly (*are they still on fire, smoldering*)?
- Any signs of a chemical powder that is causing the burn: did you brush it off and document it?

- Using the rule of 9's, determine the percentage of burn surface area (BSA).
- Were any body parts burned that are considered automatically critical (*eyes, ears, hands, feet, genitals*)?
- Did you need to activate air transport? If so, were they available? Absolutely document if you wanted air transport and they were unavailable!
- Are there any signs of swelling, especially the airway?
- Is there the presence of eschar or charred bone, blisters?
- Document the patient's pain level.
- Thoroughly document all interventions, time, who performed and the outcome (*high flow oxygen, IV access with #of attempts and success, pain medications, intubation, RSI*).
- Provide justifications on where you transported patient (*burn center, closest trauma hospital, nearest hospital*).
- Did you transport the patient emergent (*code 3*) or non-emergent (*code 1*) and justify your reasons. Did patient's condition cause you to upgrade or downgrade your transport response?
- Document any metabolic or physiologic changes that your patient displays throughout transport (*02 sat continues to drop, dyspnea becomes worse, LOC starts to diminish*).

Chapter 25

Cold Related Emergencies

Upon our arrival:

- Take note of ambient conditions, including temperature and weather.
- Where is patient found?
- Is patient wearing wet clothing? Document how you got them out of their clothes, what happened to their clothes and what you did to keep them warm.

History:

- Is there any indication of how long patient has been exposed to the cold?
- Note what the patient was wearing and if it seems appropriate for the weather or conditions the patient was found.
- Can patient or witness tell you how they found got themselves into this situation?
- Does the patient have a cardiac history?
- Is there any psychiatric history that might be a cause for this type of exposure?
- Does the patient have a history of dementia or Alzheimer 's disease?

Medications:

- Does patient take any significant medications that might lead you to a specific differential diagnosis?
- Is patient compliant with their medications?

Social:

- Any drugs or alcohol involved with this medical event?

Physical Assessment:

- What is patient's mentation upon your arrival?
- If they are unresponsive, note the time spent checking for a pulse (*is acceptable to palpate for longer than 10 seconds in this circumstance*).
- Place patient on Cardiac Monitor and note initial rhythm.
- If you are working a code, be sure to treat the patient gently and note that somewhere on your documentation.
- If possible get an axial or core temperature for your patient q 5 minutes if necessary.
- Note the temperature of your ambulance and if possible turn up the heat, noting this as well in your chart.
- Get a BGL!
- Get the patient out of their clothes in order to perform both a rapid and then detailed physical assessment looking for signs of poor circulation

and frost bite. Note how what you used to keep your patient covered throughout transport.

- Document extensively what methods you used to attempt rewarming your patient (*heat packs, layered blankets, warmed IV solutions, etc...*).

Chapter 26

Drowning/Near Drowning

Upon our arrival:

- Is this a fresh water or salt water incident?
- What is the ambient temperature?
- What is the temperature of the water (*cold, hot, ice on water*)?
- Is this a swimming pool? When was the last time it was cleaned?
- Is this a diving accident?
- Does patient have any comorbidities that could affect resuscitation efforts (*morbidly obese, diabetes, COPD, CHF*)?

History:

- When was patient last seen out of the water and conscious?
- How long was the patient submerged?
- What happened prior to the events leading up to the incident?
- Was this a boating accident? Is there trauma involved (*backboard and c-collar*)?
- Are there additional injuries?
- Was CPR or first aid started prior to EMS arrival? Document who and what was performed.

Medications:

- Any medications that the patient is taking or not taking that can help with resuscitation efforts?

Social:

- Any drugs or alcohol involved prior to incident?

Physical Assessment:

- Is this a cardiac arrest?
- What is patient's level of consciousness (*unconscious and unresponsive, disoriented, alert*)
- Note the patency of the patient's ABC's and if any management is required (*inability to protect airway, vomit, pulmonary edema*).
- Lung sounds (*rales, wheezing, rhonchi*)
- Cyanosis present?
- Initial cardiac rhythm and if shocks are administered (*what joule setting*).
- Remove wet clothing and warm patient up (*note temperature if possible and where it was taken: axillary, oral, rectal*).
- Get a BGL!
- Head to toe looking for any occult injuries.
- Note any interventions that are performed and who administered them (*IV, intubation, CPR, defibrillation*).

Chapter 27

Falls

Upon our arrival:

- Note condition of the scene to look for any possible reasons why someone fell (*icy sidewalk, cluttered house, uneven road, pot holes, spilled liquid on the ground*)
- Try to ascertain the height from which patient fell.
- Was this a fall from a standing position, were they standing on something (*chair, ladder*) or on top of something (*roof, vehicle, scaffold*).
- What did patient land on (*grass, soft dirt, sand, gravel, pavement*)?
- Document in what position the patient landed (*supine, prone, left lateral recumbent*)?
- Did patient strike feet first and then fall to their current position?
- How long were they laying there after fall.
- Were they ambulatory after fall.

History

- Did patient fall because of a syncopal episode?
- Was the patient having a medical episode prior to fall (*shortness of breath, chest pain*)?
- Is the patient diabetic?

- Does patient have a cardiac history?
- Does patient remember falling and what caused the fall?
- Did patient have sensation of vertigo prior to fall?
- Does patient have any inner ear problems?
- Has patient been losing their balance or having feelings of vertigo prior to today's fall?
- Was the patient knocked unconscious?
- Did someone or something cause them to fall following an assault?
- Has patient recently started a new diet?
- What is the ambient temperature, if hot is patient sweating or is their skin dry?

Medications:

- Is patient compliant with all of their medications?
- Has patient recently started any new medications?
- Have they recently stopped taking any medications?

Social:

- Any alcohol intake prior to fall?
- Does patient suffer withdrawals after stopping alcohol intake?
- Does patient use illicit drugs (*narcotics, hallucinogens, stimulants*)?

Physical Assessment

- What is patient's mental status as you arrive on scene (awake and oriented, unconscious, stupor, delirious, diminished)?
- Note that you took c-spine precautions and who provided in-line neck stabilization.
- Assessing the ABC's are there any problems that need to be immediately addressed, do not move on until all primary survey life threats have been managed to the best of your ability.
- Lung sounds (*clear and equal, diminished or absent, rales, rhonchi*).
- Document the full head to toe assessment looking for any occult injuries (DCAP-BTLS).
- If unstable pelvis noted, clearly document how you got patient from the ground to the backboard and to your gurney (*scoop stretcher, pelvic binder*).
- Document all procedures and note who administered them (*backboard, splint, IV, analgesia, oxygen*).
- Note any changes in mentation and the time in which they occurred throughout transport.

Chapter 28

Gunshot Wounds/Stabbings

Upon our arrival:

- Document the need for scene safety and document if you are required to stage (*make note of time you stage, time you are cleared to go in and the time you actually arrive on scene*).
- Who has possession of the weapon?
- Be as specific as you can when describing the weapon was that has been used in the assault (*6" kitchen knife vs knife, 38. Caliber pistol vs gun, approximately 7" ice pick vs sharpened object*).
- Make note of any other signs of violence when you arrive on scene (*broken bottles, blood splatters, smashed furniture*).
- Is there more than one patient?
- Is your patient violent or is there a possibility for the need to have them restrained?
- Is your patient in police custody? Do not forget to note which officer, or which police department official, is following you to the hospital.
- Is police requesting that you keep patient handcuffed throughout transport? If so, does this follow your local protocols, or will patient need to be restrained with soft restraints?

- **More than likely on these types of calls, you will not be on scene for very long, so try to make as many mental notes as you can regarding the scene before you leave.**

History:

- Most of your history will be obtained en route to the hospital. Careful documentation and time management should be noted in order to show that you provided rapid transport to the hospital.
- What was the nature of this call (*assault resulting in a shooting, sexual assault resulting in a stabbing, armed robbery resulting in attempted homicide*)? Be as specific and descriptive as you can when documenting what happened; however do not guess as to the motive of the crime. Any description you document should be attributed to someone (*police, witness, criminal suspect, patient*).
- Were any first aid or resuscitation efforts started prior to EMS arrival?

Medications:

- Does your patient take any prescription medications that might help you list potential comorbidities (*hypertension, cardiac problems, respiratory issues, diabetic*)?

Social:

- Has the patient taken any illicit narcotics prior to incident that might hamper our efforts (*opioids, stimulants, hallucinogens*)? Could make patient's statements unreliable, or the patient may present with delirious or bizarre behavior.
- Is alcohol a factor, it can mask pain and make the patient an unreliable narrator for the events that occurred. Document the presence of possible ETOH intoxication (*slurred words, bloodshot watery eyes, odor coming from patient's breath, patient admitting to consuming alcohol prior to events*).

Physical Assessment:

- Your goal is to be off the scene within ten minutes! Document time at patient's side and time you transport.
- Check life status: is patient exsanguinating? Do they have a pulse and are they spontaneously breathing?
- Manage any life threatening bleeds and the ABC's before anything else is done.
- If patient has been shot in the back, chest, abdomen or head, they should have c-spine precautions taken. Document this if it is performed.
- Patient will absolutely need to be exposed prior to being placed on a backboard.
- Perform a rapid head to toe assessment and take a careful inventory of the number of defects you

find. Remember, you are searching for the occult injuries you might not have immediately noticed, not the obvious ones that are presenting themselves to you.

- Be assured that you have scanned the patient's posterior prior to strapping them into a backboard; you may not get another chance to access this.
- Begin trending vital signs as soon as you can once en route.
- If the patient still has the penetrating object lodged inside them, document who stabilized it and how in what manner.
- Document all procedures and interventions performed during transport along with who did them and how the patient responded (intubation, IV, fluid bolus, occlusive dressing, wound care and management, ECG, 12-lead, CPR, defibrillation).
- Notify the hospital early and if applicable to your local protocols, activate a **Trauma Alert**. Be sure to timestamp when you do this as early notification is a very appropriate intervention by EMS that should be documented in your chart.

Chapter 29

Heat Related Emergencies

Upon Our Arrival:

- Note the ambient temperature and if possible humidity.
- Is there a scene safety issue?
- Where is patient found (*outside, locked car, overheated house*)?

History:

- What was patient doing at time of emergency (*exercise, working outdoors, sleeping*)
- Does patient appear to be wearing clothes that are appropriate for the weather and activity?
- How long has patient been overheated?
- Was there any change in mentation prior to EMS arrival?
- Have there been any complaints of nausea/vomiting or diarrhea?
- Has the patient been complaining of any flu-like symptoms or have they been recently febrile?

Medications:

- Any recent changes to medications?
- Has patient been taking any antipyretics (*Tylenol*)?

Social:

- Does patient have a history with taking narcotics that might cause a heat emergency (*cocaine, methamphetamines, jimson weed, Ecstasy/Molly*)?
- Is there any chance that patient might have been poisoned or had someone slip something into their food or drink (*date with a stranger, attending a party with strangers*)?

Physical Assessment:

- What is patient's mentation (*is this baseline normal or is has it acutely changed*)?
- Skin presentation (*flushed/ pale, skin turgor poor/good, furrowed tongue, still producing perspiration or are they dry/ sunken fontanelles*)
- Assess temperature
- Note condition of clothes (*dry/wet/soaked*)
- Note cooling procedures (*cold packs behind neck, axial and in groin, air conditioning in ambulance, IV fluids*).

Chapter 30

Motor Vehicle Accidents

Upon our arrival:

- En route try to think of what additional resources you might need based on the location of the event and the particulars provided by dispatch (*police- traffic control, fire/rescue- extrication, rural/remote area- rotor wing air transport*).
- It's better to get the helicopter in the air and on their way then to wait. You can always cancel them once you have gotten there, however the time you may save by launching them early could be potentially lifesaving.
- This is especially true if you got reports of serious/potentially life threatening injuries, for example: **A rollover with ejection, A patient who has been launched through the front windshield, Reports of a vehicle that rolled over a patient, Prolonged extrication required.** Once you have arrived on scene you can then determine the status of your patient and decide if you want to keep helicopter coming in or cancel them.
- Documenting scene safety is extremely important! You should briefly describe how you positioned your ambulance once you have

arrived on scene. Where you positioned the engine once it arrived on scene, hopefully it was placed in front of the accident and your ambulance.

- If you are forced to close down a street, road or highway, for safety reasons, note the direction and number of lanes you closed down and how you did it. If you provided a person to do traffic control, document it.
- How many vehicles were involved and how many patients? Multi-vehicle MVA's have the potential to quickly become an MCI.

History:

- Once on scene: do a 360' of the vehicles involved in the MVA. What parts of the vehicle were damaged (*rollover, driver side T-bone, passenger side T-bone, head-on, rear end*)? Was there any intrusion into the driver or passenger compartment?
- Was patient wearing a seat belt?
- What is the posted speed where the accident occurred?
- Do you see any tire skid marks?
- If this is a single vehicle accident: what caused it (*animal in the road, distraction with phone/radio, fell asleep*)?
- Was there a possible medical emergency that caused the traumatic event (*hypoglycemia, myocardial infarction, airway obstruction*)?

- Did vehicle come equipped with airbags and did the collision cause them to deploy?

Medications:

- Does the patient take any medications that might help lead you to learn more about possible comorbidities?
- Is patient compliant with medications?
- Are there any medications that your patient might be taking that could mask pain response or mislead a first responder about the severity of the situation (*beta blockers, pain killers*)?

Social:

- Does patient appear to be intoxicated or under the influence? While this is not our job to make this determination, we can document signs and symptoms that we observe to substantiate our suspicions (*Patient displayed slurred speech, had bloodshot watery eyes, odor of ETOH coming from his person, empty beer and whiskey bottles in vehicle, patient admits to drinking 2 beers before driving*). Remember, we are there to provide assistance, not pass judgement. This patient requires professional medical assistance, just like any other person in an emergency!
- Are there any signs and symptoms of illicit drug use (*pinpoint pupils, syringes in car, track marks*)? Take care to remember that any symptoms that might normally be associated

with narcotic use: bizarre behavior, slow or erratic breathing, diminished LOC, could also be brought on by the trauma incurred during the accident.

Physical Assessment:

- Where is your patient located (*secured by a seat belt in driver seat, thrown approximately 40' from the vehicle, slumped over the wheel unresponsive*)?
- If patient was thrown, document what they landed on (*concrete, pavement, grass, on a fence*) and in which position they were found (prone, supine, left lateral recumbent).
- Life status check, does patient show signs of life as you approach? Are there signs of obvious death (*decapitation, apneic with brain matter exposed*)?
- Who is designated to hold c-spine, were they required to be in the vehicle with patient?
- Was there any starring of the windshield? This may be a pertinent point if patient states that they were seat belted in at the time of the crash.
- Any signs of life threatening hemorrhage that needs to be addressed? How was it treated (*tourniquet, direct pressure*)?
- Is the patient's airway patent or does it manually have to be opened? Do they require suctioning?

- Breathing rate, depth and quality, are lung sounds present or do they present diminished or absent? Does your patient require supplemental oxygen or positive pressure ventilation?
- How was the patient taken out of the vehicle, or picked up off of the street?
- Patient should be exposed and a rapid head to toe assessment conducted looking for obvious and occult injuries, taking care of immediate life threats.
- The goal of any serious traumatic event is to assess, package and transport your patient within the "Platinum Ten Minutes." This starts the moment you get on scene and stops the moment you initiate transport. If you exceed this amount of time on scene you should carefully document the reasons why.
- All interventions and the person who performed them should be time stamped and documented (*supplemental oxygen, physical assessment, vital signs, neuro check pre and post securing the patient to a backboard, IV, fluid bolus, ECG, 12 lead, positive pressure ventilation, CPR, defibrillation*).
- If warranted contact the hospital as soon as you can and call a "Trauma Alert" in order to get them prepared. Document that you initiated this as this is an important part of the overall patient care you provide.

Conclusion

Practice and repetition will certainly help you towards your goal of being able to construct a strong EMS chart. However, more than simply skill you can work on and master, it has to be a goal that you really wish to obtain and are willing to put in the time and effort to accomplish that goal. The good news is it is a collection of abilities and skills you start to develop the moment you make the decision that you want to become a first responder.

EMS will always be an odd mixture of raw basic medical skills mixed in with the intuition of a provider being asked to manage an emergency while at the same time using finesse and charisma to instill confidence and provide comfort to the patient they are treating.

Your chart is the summation of this amazing skill set and an honest representation of what you are capable of accomplishing as a first responder.

Thank you so much for taking the time to read this book. I hope it has given you a deeper understanding of the responsibility you assume each time you sit down to put your words on paper, not just to your patient, but also to yourself and the profession you have chosen as a career. It is also my hope that you take away some of my enthusiasm and awe for the power and influence of the written word. To be sure, there will be a few calls that will live in your memory forever, but for the majority of your calls, they will begin to fade into your subconscious the moment you turn your patient over to the ER staff.

It is for these patients, each one hurt, sick or scared enough to activate 911, that we owe the time, attention and skill necessary to put their story down on paper.

Don't let their story slip into obscurity.

Always remain vigilant and continue to be an advocate for your patient by being perceptive while documenting each scene, meticulous in detailing what was said, and thorough in reporting what was done.

Memories may fade, but the written word can last forever.

Helpful Terminology

A

Abandonment: Termination of care without the signed consent of the patient refusing care or transferring care to a medical professional who is of equal or higher licensure.

Abduct: Movement away from the midline

Abrasion: traumatic scraping of layers of skin

Abscess: A raised area of inflamed tissue often surrounding a boil of blood or pus

Acidosis: Anything below 7 on the pH scale, however, normal pH for a human is 7.35-7.45, so blood gasses that are below 7.35 would be considered acidotic.

Acute: sudden, rapid onset

Adduction: movement towards the midline

Afebrile: without fever, normal temperature

Affect: describing a patient's demeanor or mood

Agonal: Gasping respirations that are not indicative of adequate respiration. Often seen just before a person goes into cardiac arrest.

Alkalosis: Anything that is above 7 on the pH scale, however normal pH for a human is 7.35-7.45, so blood gasses that are above 7.45 would be considered alkalotic.

Amenorrhea: without/absent menstruation

Amnesia: Loss of memory, either through a progression of advanced age, pharmaceutical medications, illicit drug use, alcohol abuse "blacking out," or from some type of psychological/ physical traumatic event.

Amputation: Loss of an appendage or limb from either a surgical procedure or traumatic event

Analgesia: Any medication or illicit drug that is taken for relief of pain. Has the high potential for dependency and abuse.

Anemia: inadequate amount of oxygen transporting material (red blood cells/hemoglobin) in a given volume of blood

Anesthesia: lacking sensation, the absence of sensation, caused by a neurological disorder, psychological disorder, pharmaceutical, or traumatic event

Aneurysm: Abnormally dilated/thinning portion of an artery that bulges and has the ominous possibility of rupturing. Can be congenital or caused by stresses such as chronic hypertension

Anorexia: Without appetite, sometimes a psychological disorder known for the patient refusing to eat due to a body dysmorphia.

Anterior: Pertaining to the front of the patient's body

Anuretic: The patient's inability to urinate.

Aphasic: The patient's inability to speak.

Apnea: Not breathing or the absence of breathing.

Arachnoid Mater: Is one of the three layers of membranes called meninges. It is the middle layer, the dura mater being the outermost and the pia mater being the innermost layers and is the site where CSF flows. The arachnoid mater surrounds the brain and the spinal cord.

Arthritis: The inflammation of a joint.

Articulation: the area where two bones are connected by a joint

Artifact: Interference that can be seen on an EKG reading preventing an accurate interpretation of the patient's cardiac rhythm.

Ascites: Accumulation of fluid in the abdominal cavity

Asphyxiation: The state or process of being deprived oxygen.

Aspirate: the inhalation of foreign objects into the airway. Usually it's food, saliva or vomitus.

Asthma: Narrowing or inflammation of the airways caused by an over response to an irritant or allergen.

Asystole: EKG "flatline", without electrical conduction/contraction

Ataxia: Absence or loss of coordination

Atrophy: A reduction in size or a wasting away of muscle and other body tissues that can be caused by malnutrition, loss of nerve supply to tissue, poor circulation and disuse/inactivity over an extended period of time.

Aura: A sensory perception that can precede a seizure allowing the patient to have an advance warning.

Auscultation: A portion of the physical assessment performed by listening, usually by stethoscope.

Autonomic Nervous System: The portion of the nervous system that controls body functions without requiring conscious thought. It can be further broken down into the **sympathetic** (fight or flight) and the **parasympathetic** (feed or breed).

Avulsion: Segment of skin or tissue traumatically cut or torn away

Axillary: The area of the body associated with the armpit.

B

Bandage: Any material that can be used to secure a dressing or a splint in place

Barotrauma: Physical damage that is caused by changes in ambient air or water pressure such as incurred while flying or diving

Battle's Signs: Is a discoloration over the mastoid process (behind the ears) that appears to be a bruise or ecchymosis that is a sign that indicates the possibility of a basilar skull fracture.

Bends: Also known as Diver's Disease, is a term used by divers that describes dissolved gasses moving out of a solution forming bubbles inside the body upon depressurization. Extremely painful with the potential for paralysis or death.

Bifurcation: Anything that can divide into two branches.

Bilateral: Something that refers to both sides, ex. *"The patient displayed equal bilateral grip strength."*

Blanch: the loss of color, ex. *"The patient's capillary bed blanched appropriately when his fingernail was compressed."*

Bloody Show: Any vaginal discharge of blood and mucus that signals the onset of labor.

Bolus: Any specified amount of fluid that is delivered by the intravenous route, usually used to meet or maintain hemodynamic status.

Bounding: Exceptionally or unexpectedly strong, usually used in reference to a patient's pulse.

Bradycardia: Relative term used for a slow heart rate, usually below 60 beats per minute. However this is dependent on the patient and the situation as people who regularly engage in cardiovascular exercise as well as trained athletes will have a normally bradycardic heart rate.

Bradypnea: Slow respirations, usually indicative of anything below 12 breaths per minute.

Breech Birth: The malpresentation during vaginal delivery in which the baby's buttocks or feet are the first to appear.

Bruit: Is an abnormal vascular sound caused by turbulent flow of blood in an artery due to either partial obstruction due to atherosclerosis or unusually high flow through an unobstructed vessel.

Buccal: Pertaining to the cheek, particularly the oral mucosa.

C

Carbon Dioxide: (CO_2) A colorless, odorless gas that is the byproduct of aerobic metabolism and which a waveform can be viewed through capnography.

Carbon Monoxide: (CO) A colorless, odorless, toxic gas produced by the inefficient oxidation of carbon compounds. It has an affinity to binds to hemoglobin approximately 200 times more than that of oxygen, causing hypoxia and possible death.

Cardiac/Cardi(o): Pertaining to the heart

Cardiomegaly: Medical terminology for an enlarged heart.

Carina: Anatomical structure where the trachea bifurcates into the left and right main stem bronchi in the lungs.

Carcinoma: An umbrella term to indicate any malignant tumor associated with cancer.

Carpopedal Spasm: A sudden and involuntary contraction of the hands, fingers, thumbs, feet and toes. Often seen by patients who are hyperventilating due to low levels of CO_2 which results in lower levels of ionized calcium and phosphate. Patients also complain of numbness and a sensation of "tingling" in their hands and feet. Situations usually remedy themselves once patient begins to breathe at a normal rate.

Cellulitis: a bacterial infection of the skin that causes inflammation and often times pain. It usually is seen as a red patch of skin with boarders that is not clearly defined which feels warm or hot to the touch. It commonly increases in size and will eventually cause cellular breakdown without antibiotic treatment.

Central Nervous System: (CNS) The brain and the spinal cord.

Cervical Spine: Consists of the first 7 vertebrae found at the base of the head and down through the neck. The first cervical vertebrae is called the atlas and the second vertebrae is called the axis. Smaller and more fragile than the rest of the spine, the cervical spine is often the site of neck pain and when injured the cause of disablement, paralysis and death.

Cholecystectomy: The surgical removal of the gallbladder.

Cholecystitis: The inflammation of the gallbladder.

Chronic: An ongoing problem or disease process.

Clonic: The abnormal jerking or alternating contraction/relaxation of muscles. Usually seen in people who suffer with a seizure disorder such as epilepsy.

Coagulation: The chemical process by which a fluid, in most circumstances blood, changes from a liquid to a solid or semi-solid state. It is part of the normal body's function to maintain homeostasis by preventing further blood loss.

Coccyx: Commonly referred to as the tailbone, it is the final segment of the vertebral column.

Cognitive: The ability to acquire knowledge and understanding through thought, experience and the use of the five senses: *touch, smell, taste, sight and hearing.*

Coma: A level of unconsciousness from which a person cannot be aroused regardless of the stimulus.

Congenital: Refers to anything that is present at birth. Commonly used in reference to certain mental/physical traits, deformities or anomalies.

Conjunctiva: A mucous membrane that lines the inside of the eyelid and covers the sclera (white of the eye).

Constrict: To make smaller or to narrow the diameter of something, i.e. *vasoconstrict.*

Cornea: Transparent tissue covering the pupil of the eye.

Cravat: A strip or roll of gauze or bandage that can be wrapped around a part of the body. Can also be formed into a triangle bandage for use as a sling.

Crepitus: The grating or popping felt and heard when two rough surfaces under the skin are rubbed together.

Crowning: The appearance of the fetus at the vaginal orifice during the second stage of birth.

Cyanosis: The bluish hue or discoloration seen on the skin or mucosa that is the result of hypoxia.

Cyst: A pocket of cells that clusters together to form a sac which contains fluid (pus/blood), air, or other contents (foreign material/debris).

D

DCAP-BTLS: Common acronym for trauma assessment. Means: *Deformities, Contusions/Crepitus, Abrasions, Punctures, Burns, Tenderness, Lacerations, and Swelling.*

Debridement: The medical removal of dead, damaged or infected tissue to improve the healing potential of the remaining skin.

Decerebrate Posture: A sign of severe injury to the brain, it is an abnormal body posture in which the body shows signs of a stiff posture where the arms and legs are extended straight out, hands open, toes pointed down and the head and neck arched backwards.

Decompression Sickness: A syndrome that occurs when a rapid decrease in ambient pressure allows nitrogen dissolved in body tissue to return to its gaseous state. Also known as "The Bends."

Decontaminate: To remove or neutralize any harmful or dangerous material from a scene or area in order to minimize the potential threat.

Decorticate Posture: A sign of severe brain injury, it is an abnormal body posture in which the body becomes rigid with arms flexed in towards body, hands closed. Not to be confused with decerebrate posturing, which is generally considered to be a more severe sign of damage.

Decubitus Ulcer: Also known as "bed sores" it is a breakdown of skin and underlying tissue due to continuous pressure on one specific body area.

Deep: Anatomical term that refers to anything that is away from the surface or the opposite of superficial.

Degenerative: A process in which the cells begin to deteriorate from their normal condition affecting the performance and efficiency of corresponding organs and tissues.

Dehydrate: The removal or loss of fluids, primarily water, from the body causing a metabolic disruption that can affect the cells, tissues or organs.

Delirious: A disruption in the thought process or ability to think clearly with a reduced awareness for the surrounding environment. It usually is associated with an acute onset of symptoms.

Delirium Tremens: A rapid onset of confusion or thought process resulting from the withdrawal of alcohol. This condition can also result in visual and auditory hallucinations, fever, diaphoresis, tremors and seizures which could result in the patient's death.

Delusion: A belief or conviction that cannot be substantiated by fact or rational argument.

Depressant: Any medication that causes the patient to have a decrease in vital physiological activities and sensations. Often times used as a sedative or analgesic and very commonly abused for these same affects.

Depressed Skull Fracture: A condition in which the skull is traumatically fractured causing bone fragments to be displaced inward.

Depression: A mood disorder that causes a persistent feeling of sadness and loss of interest. Can manifest into physical symptoms such as insomnia, changes in appetite, lack or loss of energy, inability to concentrate, failure to thrive and suicidal ideations.

Dermatitis: Inflammation of the skin.

Dermis: The inner layer of skin tissue that contains sweat glands and hair follicles. It is found just under the epidermis and above the subcutaneous layer of tissue.

Diabetic Coma: A life threatening state of unconsciousness brought on by either a lack of insulin, leading to hyperglycemia, or a lack of glucose, leading to hypoglycemia.

Diaphoresis: A medical term used to describe excessive sweating. Can be an important sign to help indicate a serious underlying medical problem.

Diaphysis: The shaft portion of a long bone.

Diarrhea: The voiding of watery stools. Can be a serious indicator of dehydration or metabolic acidosis.

Diffuse: The inability to specify a specific point of origin. Generalized and non-specific.

Dilation: To make the diameter of a vessel larger or wider.

Diplopia: Double vision.

Dislocation: An injury that occurs when two bones that come together for articulation at a joint are forced from their natural position.

Distal: Anatomical term of position that indicates something that is farther away from a point of reference, usually the heart.

Distended: Abnormally stretched, inflated or enlarged.

Diuretic: Any substance that promotes diuresis, the increased production of urine.

Dorsal: Anatomical term pertaining to the back.

Dressing: A protective covering applied directly to the wound.

Dura Mater: The outermost of the three membranes called meninges. The middle layer is known as the arachnoid membrane and the inner most is called the pia mater. One of the main functions of the dura mater is to carry blood from the brain to the heart.

Dysfunction: Abnormal function.

Dyskinesia: A disorder pertaining to the involuntary movement of muscles, such as tics, tremors and fidgetiness. It can also pertain to disorders that involve the stiff movement of muscles or the difficulty in moving muscles.

Dysmenorrhea: Pain associated with menstruation. Commonly described as cramps.

Dysphagia: Difficulty swallowing.

Dysphasia: Difficulty or impairment of speech or verbal comprehension. Often associated with a neurological condition or brain injury.

Dysphonia: Difficulty speaking often causes by congenital abnormalities or a neurological condition that affects the vocal cords.

Dyspnea: Difficulty breathing, labored breathing or the complaint of feeling short of breath.

Dysuria: Pain associated with urination or difficulty producing urine.

E

Ecchymosis: A common medical term for a bruise, the purplish discoloration that is the result of blood vessels under the skin being broken due to a traumatic impact.

Eclampsia: A serious medical complication that begins with the onset of seizures during pregnancy. Typically it is the result of being in a state of preeclampsia which is normally associated with increasing hypertension along with swelling in the hands, face and feet from the accumulation of edema.

Ectopic Pregnancy: A serious, potentially life-threatening medical condition in which the embryo attaches outside of the uterus, often the fallopian tube. As the embryo continues to grow, it puts extreme pressure on the walls of the fallopian tube causing extreme pain, usually focused on one side of the lower abdomen. If left untreated, the growing embryo will cause the fallopian tube to rupture leading to profound hemorrhage.

Edema: Swelling caused by excess fluid in the tissues.

Effusion: The movement of fluid into an anatomical space, such as a joint (joint effusion), or into the pleura space surrounding the lungs (pleural effusion).

Electrocution: Death caused by the passage of electrical current through the body.

Embolism: The sudden blockage of a vein or artery by an embolus.

Embolus: Anything that can cause the blockage of a blood vessel. It can be thickened or coagulated blood (blood embolus), fat (fat embolus) or gas (gas embolus). An embolus travels in the blood stream until it lodges somewhere. Depending on where the embolus lodges can determine if the blockage is complete (no blood is able to get through) leading to possible infarct or partial (diminished amounts of blood are able to get through) leading to ischemia and angina.

Emesis: Another word for vomiting, the forceful expulsion of stomach contents through the mouth and nose.

Emphysema: A chronic pulmonary disease in which the alveoli in the lungs are damaged, eventually weakening and then rupturing allowing for larger pockets of air to become trapped inside the lungs that cannot be used for respiration, while at the same time reducing the remaining surface area of the lungs, decreasing the amount of oxygen that reaches the bloodstream.

Enteritis: Inflammation of the intestines.

Enucleate: To surgically or traumatically extract an eye from its orbit.

Enzyme: Proteins that act as a catalyst (accelerates chemical reactions).

Epidermis: The outermost layer of the three layers of skin, the inner layers being the dermis and the hypodermis. Provides a barrier for infection and pathogens and regulates the amount of water that is lost to the atmosphere through evaporation.

Epidural Space: The potential space that is between the layers of dura mater which exists around the brain and the spinal cord. It is a common site for analgesic injection, such as the type that might be administered during childbirth.

Epigastric Region: An anatomical region of the abdomen which is located in the upper middle region above the umbilicus.

Epiglottis: A "leaf" shaped flap of cartilage that is superior to the larynx and serves to prevent food from entering the trachea.

Epilepsy: Is a group of neurological disorders marked by seizures, abnormal brain activity and alterations in mood and behavior.

Epiphysis: The rounded end of a long bone which is the primary growth section. Also known as the growth plate.

Equilibrium: A state in which opposing forces maintain balance. The human body tries to maintain equilibrium in many ways known as homeostasis.

Eschar: The thick crust that forms over burned tissue. May impede respirations if it encircles the torso limiting chest expansion during respiration and may require a surgical intervention known as an escharotomy.

Esophagus: Part of the digestive tract that connects the pharynx to the stomach.

Estrogen: Primary female sex hormone.

Etiology: The study of causes, origins, and the reasons behind why things are the way they are.

Eustachian: Part of the auditory canal, it is a tube from the middle ear to the throat.

Evisceration: The laceration or traumatic tearing of the abdominal cavity in which the internal organs are pronounced and exposed.

Exacerbate: To increase in severity or to worsen a problem.

Expectorate: To cough or spit up phlegm or blood from the lungs.

Exsanguinate: To remove blood from the body or a limb. Can also mean bleeding to death.

Extension: The movement of a limb toward a straight position.

External: Pertaining to something found on the surface, in plain sight or found on the outside.

Extremity: One of the four limbs found on the human body; an arm or a leg.

Exudate: Seepage of fluid material, often pus, through an inflammation, injury or a wound.

F

Fainting: A temporary, self-resolving loss of consciousness that is caused by your brain not receiving enough oxygen. Also known as syncope, there are several reasons for this to occur including, hypotension, vasculitis, witness to an unpleasant or shocking image, and vagus nerve stimulus.

Fallopian Tubes: The hollow tubes that connect the ovaries to the uterus.

Fascia: A layer of dense fibrous connective tissue that is found under the skin that stabilizes encloses and separates muscles and internal organs.

Febrile: Also known as a fever is typically anything that has to do with an abnormally high temperature.

Femur: The bone found in the upper leg, the thigh bone, it is the longest and strongest bone in the human body.

Fetal: Pertaining to the fetus.

Fetus: The unborn offspring of a person that has developed from an embryo.

Fibrin: A fibrous protein that is used in the production of a blood clot.

Fibula: The smaller of the two bones found in the lower leg.

Fistula: An abnormal connection between two hollow spaces, such as blood vessels, intestines and hollow organs. Sometimes seen in patients with chronic kidney problems who require dialysis. They have a surgically created arteriovenous fistula created.

Flaccid: Limp, without muscle tone.

Flail chest: The separation of a segment of ribs from the sternum producing a free moving portion of the rib cage. This free moving section is usually seen as displaying paradoxical movement, as the patient breaths in, the majority of the rib cage expands, and the free moving segment is drawn in. And as the patient breaths out, the majority of the rib cage relaxes and is drawn in, as the free segment goes the opposite way and is pushed out. Typically the result of significant blunt trauma to the chest.

Flexion: The bending of a joint.

Follicle: A canal through the skin that contains a hair.

Fontanelles: An anatomical feature found in the skull of an infant, it is the soft spaces found between the bones in the skull of an infant. At birth the infant's skull is not fully fused together allowing the skull to compress in order to pass through the vaginal opening. The fontanelles begin to close starting at 2 months and usually completely close by the time the patient turns 2 years old.

Foramen Magnum: A natural opening through a body structure. The foramen magnum is the opening at the base of the skull where the spinal cord leaves the cranial cavity.

Fossa: A hollow or depressed area below the level of the surrounding tissue.

Formed Elements: Parts of the blood composed of red and white blood cells and platelets. Red blood cells make up approximately 95% of the formed elements found in blood.

Frontal: Anatomical term pertaining to the forehead.

Frost Nip: Superficial tissue freezing.

Frostbite: Deep tissue or full thickness freezing of tissue.

Fulminant: Anything that has a sudden onset and escalates rapidly with an intensity and severity that can be lethal. Several diseases are described with this adjective such as Ebola and the bubonic plague. It can also pertain to traumatic events such as exsanguination after being shot in the chest with a gun, or the tearing of the descending aorta following an MVA.

G

Gait: The manner of walking by foot. An abnormal gait might be described as staggered, unsteady, ataxic, uncoordinated, waddling or spastic.

Gangrene: Refers to the death of tissue either due to lack of blood flow caused by illness or injury or can be the result of a serious bacterial infection.

Gastric: Pertaining to the stomach and part of the gastrointestinal tract.

Gastroenteritis: Inflammation of the stomach and intestines.

Genital: Pertaining to the sexual reproductive organs.

Genu: Hinge point connecting the femur with the tibia/fibula and protected in front by the patella. Commonly referred to as pertaining to the knee.

Geriatric: The branch of medicine that studies the problems and diseases that come with old age and the treatment of aging people.

Gestation: The period of fetal development.

Gingiva: The soft tissue surrounding the teeth, commonly referred to as gums.

Glaucoma: A medical condition characterized by abnormally high pressure in the eye. Can lead to permanent blindness.

Glottis: The true vocal cords and the space between them. This is the location where an endotracheal tube is passed during intubation.

Glucosuria: The excretion of sugar in the urine.

Goiter: Abnormal enlargement of the thyroid gland.

Gonad: The reproductive gland. In males the gonad is called the testicle and it produces sperm, in females, the gonad is called the ovary and it produces an ovum or egg.

Gout: A disorder caused by excess uric acid in the body characterized by painful joints, usually the big toe.

Grand Mal: A type of seizure, also known as a generalized tonic-clonic seizure, is the result of abnormal electrical activity in the brain causing violent muscle contractions and spasms.

Gravid: Pregnant. Often used in reference to Para/Gravida which means how many times have you been pregnant (gravida) and how many live births did you actually deliver (para).

Guarding: Protective withdrawing reaction to the actual or expected palpation of a painful or injured part of the body, usually used in reference to the abdomen.

Gynecomastia: Excessive development of the male breast tissue.

H

Hallucination: A sensory perception that is not based in reality.

Hallucinogen: A drug or medication that has the potential to stimulate hallucinations.

Hallux: Anatomical term for the big toe.

Hematemesis: The act of vomiting blood.

Hematoma: An abnormal collection of blood that has seeped out of the blood vessel wall and into the surrounding tissue. Can be caused by injury or disease and can result in significant swelling as blood continues to accumulate.

Hematuria: Blood in the urine.

Hemiplegia: An abnormal condition of being paralyzed on one side of the body.

Hemolysis: Destruction of red blood cells.

Hemophilia: A hereditary blood disorder that interferes with coagulation.

Hemoptysis: The process of coughing up blood or blood tinged sputum from the larynx, trachea or lungs.

Hemorrhage: Bleeding or the abnormal flow of blood outside of the circulatory system.

Hemostasis: The process of stopping bleeding or keeping blood inside of a damaged blood vessel.

Hemothorax: An abnormal accumulation of blood within the plural cavity between the chest wall and lungs.

Hepatitis: Inflammation of the liver tissue.

Hepato: Medical root word pertaining to the liver.

Hepatomegaly: Enlargement of the liver.

Hernia: Protrusion of an organ or organ part through the tissue that normally surrounds it.

Hives: Also known as uticaria, these are raised bumps or welts that are itchy in nature and often surrounded by reddened skin. Hives can be caused by a number of things such as allergic reaction to food, pet dander, or by the sting /bite of an insect.

Homeostasis: A self-regulating process of maintaining internal stability while adjusting to various changing conditions.

Hormone: A class of signaling molecules that are produced by glands, transported by the circulatory system in order to target distant organs to regulate physiology and behavior.

Humerus: The long bone found in the upper arm.

Hypercarbia: Excessive amounts of carbon dioxide in the body.

Hyperextension: Over extension of a body part.

Hyperglycemia: Abnormally increased concentration of glucose in the blood.

Hyperpnea: Increased depth and rate of breathing. It can be a normal response to increased exertion, or an abnormal result of a disease process such as sepsis.

Hyperthermia: Abnormally high body temperature.

Hypertrophy: The increase in size and volume of an organ or body part.

Hyperventilation: Abnormally increased rate and depth of breathing.

Hyphema: Abnormal collection of blood in the anterior chamber of the eye.

Hypocarbia: Abnormally low carbon dioxide in the blood.

Hypoglycemia: Abnormally low concentration of glucose in the blood.

Hyponatremia: Abnormally low sodium in the blood.

Hypopharynx: The distal portion of the pharynx.

Hypothermia: Abnormally low body temperature.

Hypoventilation: Abnormally low rate and depth of breathing.

Hypovolemia: A decrease in the amount of volume throughout the circulatory system. Hypovolemia can be the result of either a decrease in blood caused by trauma or internal hemorrhage, (GI blood loss) or by a decrease in salt and water (dehydration).

Hypoxemia: An abnormally low level of oxygen in the blood.

Hypoxia: An abnormal condition where the body or a portion of the body is deprived of adequate oxygen supply.

Hysterectomy: The surgical removal of the uterus.

I

Idiopathic: A disease that arises suddenly or from an unknown cause or origin.

Ileum: The portion of the small intestine located between the jejunum and the cecum.

Iliac: Superior portion of the hip bone.

Impaction: Solidly or firmly packed, often times used in reference to a blockage, such as an impaction of the bowels.

Impaled: To pierce with a sharpened object.

Impetigo: Bacterial skin infection characterized by crusted, weeping lesions.

Impotent: An erectile dysfunction that means the inability for a male to have sexual intercourse due to being unable to achieve an erection.

Incipient: Pertaining to an early stage of existence.

Incision: A cut or wound made by a sharp instrument.

Infarction: Tissue death caused by a reduced or complete blockage of blood flow, typically from an embolism or thrombosis, resulting in an inadequate oxygen supply.

Infection: The invasion of a pathogenic organism, such as bacteria or a virus, into a host's body tissues causing illness, disability or death.

Infectious: Someone who is capable of causing or transmitting an infection.

Inferior: Anatomical term relating to something that is towards the feet.

Ingestion: The act or process of taking a substance into the mouth and having it travel through the gastrointestinal tract.

Inguinal: Something that is pertaining or related to the groin.

Insomnia: A common sleep problem that affects a person's ability to fall asleep, remain asleep or wake up earlier than intended.

Insulin: A hormone produced by the pancreas that helps to lower blood sugar.

Insulin Shock: A state of severe hypoglycemia brought on by the presence of too much insulin in the blood stream. It is commonly seen as the result of a diabetic patient taking insulin and then either overexerting themselves or forgetting to eat.

Inotropic: A drug that is used to increase the force of cardiac contractions.

Integument: Pertaining to or related to the skin.

Intercostal: The muscles found between the ribs.

Internal: Anatomical term that refers to something that is deep or away from the surface.

Intravenous: Abbreviated as IV, it refers to something that is related to or administered through a vein.

Inversion: Turning inward.

Ipsilateral: Belonging to or occurring on the same side of the body.

Iris: The portion of the eye surrounding the pupil that is colored.

Ischemia: Tissue damage due to an inadequate amount of oxygen.

Ischium: The lower portion of the hip bone.

Islets of Langerhans: The cells in the pancreas that produce insulin.

Isotonic: A fluid that has the same osmotic pressure as intracellular fluid.

J

Jaundice: A yellowish discoloration seen on the skin or in the conjunctiva of the eye that is caused by an excessive amount of bile pigments in the bloodstream. Typically a sign of dysfunction or disease process involving the liver or gallbladder.

Jejunum: The second part of the small intestine which is vital for breaking down and absorbing nutrients. It is situated between the duodenum and the ileum.

Joint: A point of articulation between two bones.

Jugular Notch: Also known as the suprasternal notch is a large depression at the top of the sternum between its articulations with the two clavicles.

Jugular Vein: The major veins that carry deoxygenated blood from the head back to the heart via the superior vena cava.

Jugular Venous Distention: An engorgement of blood in the jugular veins that causes them to bulge out. Can often be a sign of cardiovascular problems as it is typically caused by a backflow into the superior vena cava due to an ineffectual blood flow through the heart.

Junctional Rhythm: A dysrhythmia originating in the atrioventricular (AV) junction.

K

Ketoacidosis: An abnormal condition that occurs when circulating insulin is inadequate and fat is metabolized into ketones and acids.

Ketonuria: A medical condition in which ketones are present in urine.

Kussmaul Respirations: An abnormal respiratory pattern characterized by deep, fast and labored breathing caused by the body's attempt to rapidly blow off CO_2 causing respiratory alkalosis in an the body's attempt to counteract metabolic acidosis.

L

Labia: The folds of skin and mucous membranes that comprise the vulva.

Labor: The stage of pregnancy that starts with contractions of the uterus and lasts until the birth of the fetus.

Laceration: A torn or jagged wound produced by the tearing of body tissue.

Lacrimal Gland: The tear secreting gland found in the eye.

Lactation: The secretion of milk from the mammary glands.

Laparotomy: A medical or surgical incision into the abdominal cavity.

Laryngeal: Pertaining to the larynx.

Laryngeal Edema: The inflammation and swelling of the larynx commonly caused by trauma (burns, blunt force) or allergic reaction (anaphylaxis). It can quickly become a life-threatening situation if the swelling impairs oxygen from getting into and out of the lungs.

Laryngospasm: A sudden, uncontrolled constriction of the vocal cords that can prevent air from passing into the lungs.

Larynx: The voice box.

Lateral: Anatomical term referring to something towards the side and away from the midline.

Lateral Recumbent: Lying on the side.

Lateral Rotation: The turning or twisting of an extremity away from the midline.

Lavage: The process of irrigating or washing out a body cavity, such as the stomach or bowels.

Lethargy: A state of weariness, fatigue, lack of energy or profoundly feeling tired.

Leukemia: A cancer of the body's blood forming materials, including the bone marrow and lymphatic system. Usually involving the body's white blood cells (leukocytes) this cancer causes an abnormal proliferation of cells to develop which no longer function properly.

Leukocytes: White blood cells that are cells of the immune system and used to fight infections disease and foreign invaders.

Ligament: A fibrous tissue that connects bone to bone.

Ligate: To tie off a tube or a blood vessel.

Lividity: Having a bluish discoloration of the skin caused by bruising, strangulation, congestion of blood vessels or stagnation of blood flow.

Localized: Pertaining to a small or specific part of the body.

Lordosis: A condition of the spine where the lower lumbar portion curves inward resulting in the appearance of a concave back when viewed from the side.

Lucid: Having a clear meaning without the appearance of confusion.

Lumbar: The third region of the spine below the cervical and thoracic spine, these five vertebras extends from the lower rib cage to the pelvis.

Lumen: The channel or space that is found within a hollow tube, such as vein or an artery.

Lumpectomy: The surgical removal of a mass (often a malignancy) from the breast tissue without disruption of surrounding tissue.

Lupus: A systemic autoimmune disease that occurs when the body's immune system begins to attack its own tissues and organs.

Lymph: A yellowish fluid that flows through the lymphatic system. It functions to transport proteins, fats and excess interstitial fluid back to the bloodstream. This fluid may also pick up certain bacteria and deposit them in lymph nodes where they are destroyed.

Lymphangitis: An inflammation or infection of the lymphatic system which occurs as the result of an infection found at a site distal to the lymphatic channels that are affected.

Lymph Node: Kidney shaped nodes that are found throughout the body that act as filers for the lymphatic system.

Lymphoma: A malignancy found in the lymphatic system or any of its components.

M

Malaise: A general feeling of discomfort, unease or pain. Can often be a precursor to a more serious disease or infection.

Malignancy: The tendency for a medical condition to get progressively worse. Most often used as a condition of cancer in that a malignant cancer is one that is not self-limiting and has the potential to grow and spread.

Malleolus: The bony protuberance on each side of the ankle.

Malunion: A fractured bone that hasn't healed properly.

Mandible: The lower jawbone. It is the largest and strongest bone in the human face.

Manubrium: The upper portion of the sternum above the angle of Louis.

Masticate: The act of chewing.

Mastoid: The portion of the skull that lies immediately posterior to the ear.

Maxilla: The upper jawbone.

Meconium: A thick, greenish tar like substance that lines the intestines of the fetus while in utero. The presence of this during birth indicates the baby has had a bowel movement prior to birth and can be a sign of possible fetal distress.

Medial: Anatomical term for toward the midline of the body.

Mediastinum: The central portion of the thoracic cavity that contains the heart and its vessels, the esophagus, and the trachea.

Medulla Oblongata: The portion of the brain that controls vegetative functions.

Meninges: Three membranes that line the brain and spinal cord. The membranes are the dura mater, the arachnoid mater and the pia mater.

Meningitis: An inflammation of the meninges, usually from a viral infection but bacterial, parasitic and fungal infections can also cause this.

Menopause: The permanent cessation of menstrual activity.

Menorrhagia: An excessive or abnormal amount of bleeding that occurs during menstruation.

Menses: The discharge that occurs during menstruation.

Menstruation: The sloughing off of the uterine lining each month by a woman of childbearing age.

Metacarpal: The bones of the hand from the wrist to the fingers.

Metastasis: The pathological spread of a disease producing agent, such as cancer, from an initial or primary site to a secondary site.

Metatarsal: The bones of the foot from the ankle to the toes.

Midclavicular line: Anatomical term for the imaginary vertical line which begins in the middle of the clavicle and runs down the body.

Midline: Anatomical term for the imaginary vertical line that starts at the center of the body and divides it into right and left halves.

Miosis: Extreme or excessive constriction of the pupil. "Pinpoint pupils."

Miscarriage: The spontaneous loss of a pregnancy before the 20th week.

Mitral Valve: Also known as the bicuspid valve, is a one way valve found in the heart between the left atrium and the left ventricle.

Morbidity: A diseased condition or state.

Mnemonic: A series of words used to assist memorization, such as *Stupid Dogs Jump In Crap And Tell Dumb Silly Riddles:* to describe the gastrointestinal tract: *Stomach, Duodenum, Jejunum, Ileum, Cecum, Ascending, Transverse, Descending, Sigmoid, Rectum.*

Mucous Membrane: A membrane that lines many organs of the body and contains mucous secreting glands.

Multifocal: Pertaining to or coming from many different foci or locations.

Multipara: A woman who has had more than two pregnancies.

Myalgia: Pains or aches felt in the muscles of the body, often associated with extreme exertion or exercise. It can however, be a symptom of something serious such as DVT's, myocardial infarction, lupus, Lyme disease and MS.

Mydriasis: Extreme or excessive dilation of the pupil. "Blown pupils."

Myocardium: Pertaining to the heart muscle.

Myoclonus: Rapid, involuntary muscle spasm, jerk or twitch. A hiccup is an example of a myoclonus.

N

Narcolepsy: Abnormal medical condition that causes sudden and unexpected periods of sleep.

Nasopharyngeal: Pertaining the nasopharynx.

Nasopharynx: The portion of the pharynx that is found just superior to the palate.

Nausea: A diffuse and uncomfortable sensation often perceived as an urge to vomit.

Necrosis: A form of cell injury that results in the premature death of cells in living tissues.

Necrotic: Pertaining to dead tissue.

Neonatal Period: The first 4 weeks of a child's life after birth.

Neonate: A newborn usually associated with a child during their first month of life.

Neoplasm: A mass of tissue exhibiting unusually rapid growth commonly referred to as a tumor.

Nephrotoxic: Toxicity of the kidneys caused by the ingestion or buildup of chemicals or medications that can have poisonous results.

Neuralgia: A pain that passes along the distribution of a nerve.

Neurotoxic: A form of toxicity caused by a physical, chemical or biological agent that has an adverse effect on the structure or function of the central or peripheral nervous system.

Nocturia: The sensation of having to get up at night to urinate.

Nocturnal: Something that is pertaining to or occurring at night.

Nonviable: Incapable of maintaining independent existence, often referred to a premature embryo.

Nosocomial Infection: A hospital acquired infection.

Nulligravida: A woman who has never been pregnant.

Nullpara: A woman who has never given birth.

Nystagmus: A medical condition where a person has rapid involuntary movement of their eyes, often making it difficult or impossible for them to keep their eyes fixed on any specific object. May affect both eyes (bilateral) or just one eye (unilateral).

O

Obese: A medical condition in which a person's excess body fat begins to have negative health effects on their health.

Oblique: Something that is situated at an inclined position, not transverse or horizontal.

Occipital: The bone that forms the back or the skull.

Occlude: The block, obstruct or close off.

Occult: Something that is hidden or not in a place that can be obviously seen or noticed.

Ocular: Pertaining to the eye.

Olecranon Process: The large, thick portion of the ulna that forms the pointy tip of the elbow.

Oncology: Branch of medicine that deals with the diagnosis, management and prevention of cancer.

Oral: Pertaining to the mouth.

Orbits: Also known as the eye sockets, they are the cavities in the skull that hold the eyeballs.

Oropharynx: The area between the soft palate in the mouth and the epiglottis.

Orthopnea: Difficulty breathing or shortness of breath that occurs when lying down.

Orthostatic: Dramatic decrease in blood pressure when sitting down or standing up.

Osteoporosis: Abnormal medical condition when the bones in the human body become increasingly porous, causing them to become brittle and more susceptible to breakage.

Ovulation: The release of a mature ovum from the ovaries.

Ovum: A single unfertilized egg.

P

Palate: The roof of the mouth that separates the oral from the nasal cavity.

Palliative: Area of care that deals with relieving and treating the suffering of patients.

Pallor: The presence of a pale color of skin that can be the result of trauma, emotional stress or illness.

Palmar: Related to or involving the hand.

Palpate: The process of using one's hands to examine a patient.

Palpitation: The perception of feeling an abnormal heartbeat. It is usually described as a fluttering, pounding or rapid heartbeat.

Pancreas: An organ that is part of the digestive system and endocrine system that functions to regulate blood sugar in the bloodstream and aid in the digestion of food by excreting digestive juices into the small intestine.

Pancreatitis: The inflammation of the pancreas.

Paradoxical Movement: An abnormal condition that exists when the normal movement of respiration is reversed, the wall of the chest moves in during inspiration and out during expiration. It is most commonly caused by a traumatic event involving chest, specifically the rib cage.

Paralysis: The loss of sensation or motor function in one or more muscles.

Paraplegia: The loss of sensation or motor function in the lower extremities.

Parenteral: The administration of a drug or medication by means other than oral or the alimentary canal, such as intermuscular or subcutaneous injection, intravenous or interosseous.

Paresis: A condition in which movement of a muscle or muscle group has become impaired or weakened.

Paresthesia: An abnormal sensation felt on the skin without any apparent physical cause. It can be described in a number of different ways such as "pins and needles," chilling, burning or a numbing sensation.

Patella: A flat circular bone that articulates with the femur and acts to cover and protect the anterior surface of the knee joint. It is commonly referred to as the knee cap.

Patency: A term used to refer to something that is open and clear or a lack of obstruction. The word is commonly used in EMS to refer to the airway and whether the airway appears patent or not.

Pedal: Pertaining to the foot.

Pelvic Cavity: The body cavity that is surrounded by the pelvic girdle and contains the reproductive organs, the urinary bladder, the colon and the rectum.

Percussion: A means of assessment by tapping the body at various points to determine the density of the underlying structures based on the sound it produces.

Percutaneous: Anything that is administered, such as an injection, absorbed, as in an ointment or transdermal patch, or removed from the skin.

Perfusion: The process by which oxygenated blood is delivered to body tissues and deoxygenated blood is removed from body tissues.

Pericardial Effusion: Excess fluid built up or trapped within the pericardial sac.

Pericardium: A thin, double walled sac, which surrounds the heart and roots of the great vessels (vena cava and aorta). It keeps the heart lubricated, protected and helps to maintain stabilization, keeping the heart in place.

Perineum: The area of skin between the genitals and the anus.

Periorbital: Referring to around the eyeball or eye socket.

Peritoneum: The membrane that lines the abdominal cavity.

Peritonitis: The inflammation of the peritoneum.

Petechiae: Tiny red, purple or brown spots found on the skin, usually the result of minor blood vessel hemorrhages.

Petit Mal Seizure: Also called absent seizures, they are the brief, sudden lapse of consciousness which may be accompanied by involuntary muscle twitches or repetitive movement such as lip smacking or fluttering of eye lids.

Phalanx: Bones of the finger or toe. The plural of the word is phalanges.

Phantom Pain: Is the sensation of pain an amputee feels from a limb that is no longer there.

Phlebitis: Inflammation of the vein.

Phlegm: Mucus that originates from the respiratory tract.

Photophobia: Painful hypersensitivity to light.

Pica: An eating disorder which presents as an appetite for substances that are not normally considered food, such as rocks, dirt or hair.

Plantar: Relating to the bottom or the arch of the foot.

Plasma: The straw colored fluid portion of blood that does not contain red or white cells.

Platelet: Also called thrombocytes, they are an element found in the blood that is necessary for blood clotting.

Pleura: A membrane that lines the outer surface of the lungs and the inner surface of the thoracic cavity.

Pleuritis: An inflammation of the pleura.

Pneumonectomy: The surgical removal of a lung.

Pneumothorax: A partial or completely collapsed lung caused when air leaks into the space between the lung and the walls of the thoracic cavity.

Polydactyly: Congenital defect that occurs when a person has more than the normal amount of fingers or toes.

Polydipsia: An excessive thirst or an abnormal desire to intake fluids.

Polyp: An abnormal mass of tissue projected out of a mucous membrane, such as the lining of the intestines or the cervix.

Polyphagia: An abnormal hunger or appetite or the intense desire to eat.

Polyuria: An excessive or abnormally large amount of urine production.

Popliteal Fossa: The posterior aspect of the knee joint.

Posterior: An anatomical term used to indicate something towards the back.

Postictal: The altered state of consciousness that can occur immediately following a seizure. Common in patients who have been diagnosed with epilepsy and suffer seizures, the period of time a person remains postictal varies, but usually lasts between 5 to 30 minutes.

Postpartum: Something that occurs, or the period of time following childbirth, it can refer to something soon after birth, such as postpartum hemorrhage, or days to months afterwards, such as postpartum depression.

Prenatal: Something that occurs from the time a woman becomes pregnant until she is no longer carrying a fetus.

Prepubescent: The period of human development that occurs before puberty.

Priapism: Persistent abnormal erection of the penis.

Primipara: Medical term used to describe a woman's first pregnancy.

Prognosis: A medical term used to predict a patient's likely outcome based on their current standing.

Prolapsed Cord: A delivery in which the umbilical cord presents before the baby's body.

Pronation: Turning or rotation of the hand or forearm in a way so that the palm faces backwards or downwards.

Prone: Anatomical term used to describe someone who is lying face down.

Proptosis: The bulging or forward displacement of the eye from out of the orbit.

Prostate: A gland at the base of the male urinary bladder.

Prosthesis: An artificial device that is used to replace a missing body part.

Prostration: A complete mental or physical collapse or to make something extremely weak or powerless.

Protocol: A formal set of established rules or plans developed to help manage a specific medical problem or event.

Proximal: Anatomical term referring to something that is closer to a specific origin point or point of reference.

Pruritus: Itchy skin which can be caused by a number of medical conditions such as dry skin, hay fever, eczema, pregnancy and diabetes.

Ptosis: Abnormal medical condition when the top eyelid partly or completely droops down over the eye.

Puberty: The period of human development when a sexually immature child develops into a sexually mature adult.

Pulmonary: Pertaining to the lungs.

Pulsatile: Throbbing rhythmically, as with the heartbeat.

Purulent: Something that is filled with or draining pus.

Pus: A thick whitish-yellow fluid that is made up of dead white blood cells, bacteria, tissue debris which is the result of the body's attempts to fight off a bacterial or fungal infection.

Pyrexia: Also known as a fever, it is someone who displays a normal body temperature over the normal range.

Pyrogenic: Something that can cause a fever.

Pyrosis: Discomfort of a burning nature, such as heartburn or GERD, which is felt in the upper abdomen, chest or the throat.

Pyuria: Abnormal finding of pus in the urine.

Q

Quadrant: One quarter of an area, usually used to designate which aspect of the abdomen you are assessing.

Quadriplegia: The partial or complete paralysis of both the arms and legs.

Quickening: A movement, felt by the mother, of the fetus in utero.

R

Raccoon Sign (Eyes): Bilateral periorbital ecchymosis sometimes seen with a basal skull fracture.

Radius: The bone on the thumb side of the lower arm.

Rales: Also referred to as crackles, these are adventitious breath sounds heard as air moves through congested bronchioles. Often described as sounding like stands of hair being rubbed together.

Rectum: The final portion of the large intestine where feces accumulates just before it is ready to be discharged from the body.

Recumbent: Pertaining to or referring to lying horizontally.

Reduce: To move or manipulate a fractured or dislocated bone back into its normal position.

Referred Pain: Pain that is felt at a location other than where it originates.

Reflex: Involuntary contraction of a muscle by applying an external, mechanical stimulus to the muscle or tendon.

Reflux: Flow that is moving opposite the normal direction.

Regurgitation: The expulsion of material, usually undigested food or blood, from the oropharynx or nasopharynx via the esophagus.

Renal: Pertaining to the kidney.

Respiration: The exchange of oxygen and carbon dioxide between the lungs, blood and tissues.

Resuscitation: The effort to manually restore a circulating pulse and perfusing blood flow in a person who has gone into cardiac arrest.

Retina: A thin layer of tissue that lines the back of the eye near the optic nerve that converts visual images into nerve impulses.

Retractions: The use of accessory muscles such as the sternocleidomastoid and the scalene in an effort to maximize respiratory effort, usually a sign of respiratory distress.

Rhonchi: Lung sounds, which are continuous and rattling, often sounding like snoring, which are usually caused by secretions in the lungs, primarily the larger bronchial trees.

Rhinitis: Inflammation of the nasal mucosa.

Rhinoplasty: Surgical repair or elective cosmetic alteration of the nasal structure.

Rigor Mortis: The period after death when the body's muscles become stiff and rigid. How long this period lasts depends on a number of factors such as ambient heat, humidity, and if the person was suffering from a fever or infection at the time of death.

Rotator Cuff: A group of four muscles: the supraspinatus, infraspinatus, teres minor and subscapularis that surround, stabilize and allow for mobility of the shoulder joint.

S

Sacral: Pertaining to the sacrum.

Sacrum: A large triangular shaped bone at the base of the spine that fuses together the five sacral vertebrae. It is found just inferior to the lumbar spine and superior to the coccyx.

Saline: A fluid that is made up primarily from a solution of water and sodium chloride.

Scald: Burn caused by hot liquid or steam.

Scapula: Flat, triangle shaped bone that comprises the shoulder blade.

Sclera: The fibrous outer layer of the eyeball which makes up the "white" of the eye.

Sclerosis: A pathological condition that occurs when tissue or an anatomical feature has become hardened and overrun by an overgrowth of fibrous tissue or an increase in interstitial tissue.

Scoliosis: Lateral curvature of the spine.

Scrotal: Pertaining to the scrotum.

Scrotum: The external pouch of skin where the testes are located.

Sepsis: A systemic presence of infectious organisms.

Septum: An anatomical structure that divides cavities or tissue, such as in the one found in the nose or in the heart.

Sequela: Problems that follow and are caused by a disease, trauma or disorder.

Serum: The liquid portion of blood that does not play a part in clotting or coagulation.

Shock: The inadequate perfusion of tissue caused by a medical disorder or traumatic event.

Sign: A pertinent finding which can be observed on a patient during a physical assessment.

Sinus: An opening found in a bone.

Soft Palate: The muscular tissue found on the roof of the mouth at the posterior aspect.

Spasm: A sudden involuntary muscle contraction.

Sphygmomanometer: The technical term for a blood pressure cuff.

Splenomegaly: An enlarged spleen.

Sprain: Injury to the ligament surrounding a joint.

Sputum: Mucus that is coughed up from the airway or the pharynx.

Stasis: The slowing down or cessation of the flow of body fluid, usually referring to blood or urine.

Stat: A commonly used medical term meaning "immediately." It comes from the Latin word statum which is translated as "at once."

Stenosis: The abnormal narrowing of a blood vessel.

Status Asthmaticus: Severe asthmatic episode which is unresponsive to medications.

Sternal: Pertaining to the sternum.

Sternum: The bone commonly referred to as the breast bone which has a majority of the ribs attached to it and has the manubrium at the superior end and the xyphoid process at the inferior end.

Stoma: A small artificial opening.

Strain: Injury caused by the stretching of the muscle beyond its natural limits.

Stridor: High-pitched sound associated with upper airway obstruction.

Stroke: Also referred to as a cerebrovascular accident (CVA) it is the obstruction or blockage of blood flow to a part of the brain due to either an embolism or the rupture of a blood vessel.

Stupor: A diminished level of consciousness associated with confusion, lethargy or drowsiness.

Subcutaneous: Something that occurs or is administered to the layer of skin just below the epidermis.

Subluxation: Incomplete dislocation of a joint, where the bone ends remain in some partial contact.

Substernal: Anatomical reference to something felt or occurring in the center of the chest under the sternum.

Superficial: Near the surface.

Superior: Anatomical term used to denote something that is above another body part.

Supination: Turning or twisting the arm so that the palm faces upward or an inversion of the foot.

Supine: Anatomical term relating to someone who is lying on their back, face up.

Suprapubic: Lower central abdominal region above the pubis.

Symptom: A subjective complaint told by a patient.

Syncope: A brief, self-resolving loss of consciousness commonly referred to as fainting.

Syndrome: A collection of signs and symptoms that is peculiar to a specific disorder or disease process.

Synovial Fluid: The fluid that lubricates joints so that bones are able to articulate smoothly.

Systemic: Something that is affecting the body as a whole.

T

Tachycardia: Rapid heart rate above the normal limits, usually considered to be100 beats per minute. Can be the normal result of exertion, excitement or fright or it can also be pathological in nature, such as in hypovolemic, cardiogenic or septic shock.

Tachypnea: Respiration rate above the normal limits, usually considered to be around 20 breaths per minute. Can be the normal result of exertion, excitement or fright, or it can be the pathological result of disease, such as COPD, Asthma, CHF or injury, such as a tension pneumothorax, flail chest or pulmonary contusion.

Tactile: Pertaining to the sense of touch.

Tarsal: Pertaining to the ankle.

Temporal: The area of the skull located on the lower lateral sides just above the ears.

Tendon: Fibrous connective tissue that attaches muscles to bone.

Testicular Torsion: An abnormal twisting of the testicle within the scrotum.

Tetralogy: A group of four signs or symptoms that have something in common.

Thenar Eminence: The mass of tissue at the base of the thumb.

Thoracic: Pertaining to or referring to the chest.

Thrombus: A blood clot that formed inside of a blood vessel.

Thrush: A yeast-like oral infection caused by the Candida albicans fungus.

Tibia: The larger bone in the lower leg also referred to as the "shin" bone.

Tic: The sudden spasmodic twitching of a group of muscles.

Tinnitus: An abnormal ringing in the ears.

Tonic: A prolonged or persistent muscle contraction, seen commonly with people having an epileptic seizure.

Trachea: Commonly called the windpipe, it is a cartilaginous tube that connects the larynx to the lungs.

Trauma: Harmful or life threatening condition that is caused by an event, series of events or a set of circumstances that causes physiological or psychological injury.

Tragus: The cartilaginous projection located on the ear just anterior to the external auditory canal.

Trendelenburg Position: Supine with legs raised and head lowered.

Tricuspid Valve: One way cardiac valve located between the right atrium and the right ventricle that allows blood to travel in a forward flow throughout the right side of the heart and into the pulmonary valve which leads to the pulmonic artery.

Trimester: Roughly lasting 3 months, it is considered to be one-third of a pregnancy.

Trismus: A lasting spasm of the jaw muscles causing the teeth to remain clenched tightly shut. It can be a serious life threat if advanced airway management is required.

Turgor: The degree of elasticity of the skin, it is used clinically to determine the extent of dehydration or fluid loss in the body.

Tympanic Membrane: The part of the inner ear known as the eardrum.

U

Ulcer: A lesion or open sore that is found on the surface of the skin or body organ.

Ulna: The larger bone of the lower arm.

Umbilicus: Commonly referred to as the bellybutton, it is also an anatomical landmark when visualizing and examining the abdomen.

Ureter: The tubes that convey urine from the kidneys to the bladder.

Urethra: The tube that carries urine from the bladder to the urethral orifice, in men located in the shaft of the penis and in women just above the vaginal opening, below the clitoris.

Uticaria: A transient condition of the skin usually caused by an allergic reaction and characterized by itchy, irregularly elevated patches of pale or reddened hives or wheals.

Uvula: The small growth of soft tissue that hangs from the soft palate at the back of the mouth.

Uterus: The organ that holds and nourishes the fetus.

V

Vagina: The elastic, muscular canal from the uterus to the vulva.

Vallecula: The slot at the base of the tongue and posterior to the epiglottis.

Vascular: Relating to blood vessels.

Vasoconstriction: The narrowing of the diameter of a blood vessel which tends to increase resistance and the workload of the heart to force blood through, resulting in an increase in blood pressure.

Vasodilation: The increase in diameter of a blood vessel which tends to decrease resistance and lowers the workload of the heart to push blood through, typically resulting in a decrease in blood pressure.

Vein: A blood vessel that returns deoxygenated blood to the right side of the heart. The one exception is found in the circulatory system where the pulmonary vein carries oxygenated blood back to the left side of the heart from the lungs.

Venous: Pertaining to a vein.

Venule: A small blood vessel that makes up part of the microvasculature in the human body.

Vernix: The waxy, cheese like material that is typically seen on newborn just after delivery.

Vertebrae: The bones of the spinal column. There are 7 cervical vertebrae, 12 thoracic vertebrae, 5 lumbar vertebrae, 5 fused vertebrae that make up the sacrum and the small 3-5 fused vertebrae that make up the coccyx (tailbone).

Vertigo: The sensation that the surrounding area around a person is moving or spinning making them feel off-balance, nauseated and dizzy.

Viable: Capable of being kept alive.

Virulence: The ability of a pathogen to provoke a disease process in a host.

Void: The act or process of excreting waste products from the human body, such as urine or feces.

Vomit: The expulsion of gastric contents through the mouth or nose usually comprised of undigested food products or blood.

Vomitus: the material ejected from the stomach by vomiting.

W

Wheal: Area of raised skin caused by subcutaneous fluid.

Wheeze: A continuous, coarse, whistling sound heard when breathing, typically caused by a narrowing or inflammation of the airway passage. Common causes are asthma, allergic reaction and COPD.

Word Salad: The jumbled often meaningless words or phrases spoken by an individual afflicted with certain neurological or mental disorders, such as a cerebral vascular accident (CVA) or schizophrenia.

X

Xyphoid Process: The sharp arrowhead shaped protrusion located at the inferior edge of the sternum.

Z

Zygomatic Bone: Commonly called the cheek bone, it is the part of the skull that forms the inferolateral aspect of the orbit, as well as makes up a portion of the floor of the orbit.

About the Author

A 20-year veteran of EMS service, Paul Serino has made continuous professional development a lifelong goal. Getting his start in Albuquerque, New Mexico where he was fortunate to work alongside some of the world's greatest first responders and educators at Albuquerque Ambulance. In 2002, Paul and a small group of his friends convinced each other to attend paramedic school at Eastern New Mexico University in Roswell, New Mexico. It was there that Paul made the decision to focus on EMS as a career. Spending a career working as a paramedic, a firefighter, a movie set medic and EMS educator, Paul has consistently tried to strive for the highest standard of patient care. In addition, Paul has been able to merge his degree in Journalism with his passion for EMS by writing several articles for local EMS newsletters and national trade publications such as EMS World. In 2016, Paul and his family moved to Florida where he currently works as a faculty staff member with St. Petersburg College teaching EMTs and paramedic students. In addition to working Paul enjoys spending time going to Sci-Fi/Horror conventions, reading Star Wars novels and taking advantage of the numerous amusement parks found in Florida, particularly Disney World. Paul's other hobby is driving his wife and daughter crazy with essential movie trivia that they should and must know.

This is Paul's second book.

Please Review

This book has been an absolute labor of love for me and I hope you enjoyed it. However, now that you're done with it, will you please do me a favor and take the time to review this book online wherever you purchased it?

Good, bad or indifferent, I've learned to develop a tough skin along with a healthy sense of humility.

If you have suggestions or comments I would love to hear them.

Take care and always stay safe out there.

I also wanted to thank a few people who without their help I'm not certain I could have gotten this book written just the way I wanted it to turn out.

Writing a book, any book, is not an easy feat. So first and foremost, I want to thank the extraordinary amount of patience and encouragement that my wife Stacy has given me throughout this adventure. Thank you for allowing me the time necessary to sit and concentrate until I was able to type this all out.

I also would like to thank my Uber-smart friend Krista Fusari for reviewing my manuscript and helping me fine tune it into a presentable book.

And of course to Mike Buldra, who was the academic and spiritual guru to our paramedic class. It was in

Roswell that I learned just how much I loved EMS and how much respect it truly deserves. You asked us to always give you our best in the classroom, because our patients deserves our best out in the real world. It's a sentiment that I try to impart to my students every day I am with them.

You ran one hell of a show Mr. Buldra!

We've never forgotten what you taught us!

Paul Serino